Minister of Death

Mark G. Kortepeter

ALPENBLICK PUBLISHERS, EDITION APRIL 2026

A version of this book was published in 2004 under the title, "Biohazard 9-1-1." This new version has been re-written with extensive character, dialogue, plot, and scene modifications.

ISBN (print): 979-8-9956473-0-0
ISBN (ebook): 979-8-9956473-1-7

1

May 4, 1997 (DAY 0)

Jed Thorton pulled off the highway onto a dirt road and braked his rusty black Ford F-150 pickup truck. He rolled down his window and inhaled the crisp pine-scented morning air, as refreshing as the scent of clean laundry emerging from the dryer. Birds called from the surrounding woods in response to the awakening day. He put his hand to his forehead to block the morning sun that peeked over the edge of Upper Wolfjaw Mountain as he took in the beauty of the valley below. The surrounding deep pine forest was bathed in a warm yellow glow, but at the base of the valley, Glacier Lake still hid beneath a white blanket of cottony mist nestled among the shadows not yet penetrated by the sunlight.

Putting the truck back in gear, Jed bounced along as the truck coasted down the potholed dirt road, its rusting struts squeaking with each bump. The dense forest eventually opened into a large clearing on a bluff overlooking one edge of the lake. Jed pulled up near a white trailer, its weather-worn metal siding displaying patches of cancerous rust. The truck door screeched as he opened it, interrupting the serenity of the quiet valley around him.

Jed was in his early fifties, but his leathery skin from years of sun and cigarettes made him look twenty years older. It was a cold morning for May, even for New York's Adirondack high peaks, especially in the dark valley. Jed welcomed the impending warmth of the sun as the surrounding hills began to awaken in its tracks. He stood by the truck momentarily, cupped his hands to light a cigarette, then let the cigarette dangle from his lips as he stuffed his hands into his pockets to warm them.

The murmur of muffled voices broke the silence just before the trailer door squeaked open and three men emerged, their breath fogging in the morning air. One man left the others and walked over to a quiet backhoe sitting on the edge of the clearing. Moments later, the backhoe awoke and coughed out dense blue smoke, shattering the stillness in the air. Then it turned and rolled toward a trench along the edge of the lake, followed by a dust cloud.

Jed flicked his cigarette away then grabbed his lunch pail and hard hat from the bed of the pick-up. He pulled up his sagging pants and trudged toward the remaining two men. He felt the air temperature drop further as he approached them.

"Mornin' boys," Jed said. "Good to see you up an' at it."

"Hey boss," the two workers responded nonchalantly.

"We need to get a move on today," Jed said. "We're purty near done with the pipe layin', but we can't afford any more delays."

"Yeah, boss," Otis Whitman acknowledged. He was the shorter and heavier of the two and wore grimy jeans and a red-flannel shirt. "But that damn ice has been a pain in the ass."

"Yeah, yeah, I've heard enough excuses to write a book," Jed responded. "I know that ice is a bitch, but if we don't get this pipe in the ground, the big man's gonna chew my ass." Jed worried about more than the owner's wrath. Visions of overdue medical bills, a mortgage, and his nagging wife filled his thoughts. He couldn't afford to lose this job because of a little ice.

Otis frowned. "But boss…"

"No more buts. The only butts I want to see are yours, in that trench. Get that last twenty feet done by the cave. Scott can help you cut through that with the backhoe this morning. Then you can finish bulldozing the clearing." He gestured toward a partially cleared area off the side of the truck.

"Sure boss." Otis shrugged and shivered. "I hope those fancy people who stay in this hotel someday will freeze their asses off, just like us."

"Not likely, but I hear ya," Jed replied, pointing at a large cave opening close to the lake, surrounded by a pile of boulders. "It *is* kinda stupid to put it near that cave. That is the darndest thing – fills up with snow and ice all winter and acts like a 'frigerator the rest of the year. It's a great place to keep your beer cold, though."

"Yeah, but good luck finding people who want to freeze." Roger Jamison, the other worker, remarked. His skeletal thin frame showed through a torn gray undershirt and an unzipped mud-splattered utility jacket.

"Oh, they'll have no problem findin' people, on account of the trout," Jed answered. "We used to fish here when I was a kid. Used to be our local secret, but this hotel will be the end of that, when the fat cats come up here and pretend they care about the mountains."

"Yeah. Rich bastards," Roger said.

"Now check that out," Jed said, pointing at the lake. "Check out that mist floatin' out of the cave." The others watched as Jed waved his arm, imitating the pathway of the cottony mist that billowed out of the cave.

Otis and Roger nodded. "Yeah? So?" said Roger.

"Well, damn it. That's what keeps this side of the lake so cold. The trout love it. Keeps the ground cold, too. That's why we have all that ice to hack through." Jed cringed, feeling a blast of cold air on the back of his neck.

"Okay boys," Jed said abruptly. "Quit wastin' time! This hotel's our bread and butter. Now get your asses moving!"

"But boss," Roger objected, his missing front teeth showing.

"I already said no buts. Now get a move on."

"Aye aye, Sarge," Otis gave Jed a mock salute.

"Wrong military service, son. We don't use 'aye aye' in the Army. Don't mix up the Army with the Navy, or you might piss me off."

“Whatever. I’ll get the tools.” Otis said reluctantly as he walked away slowly.

"I'll just finish this here smoke and be off,” Roger said with a grin. His jeans had dried mud spattered on them, and the soles of his boots were separating from the tops. He took one long puff and flicked the cigarette over the bluff. It disappeared into the fog and made a quiet hiss as it hit the cold water. He turned to follow Otis.

"Hey," Jed called after the men. "You boys headin’ home tonight?"

"Sure boss,” Otis replied. “Got a family, ya know."

"Yeah, yeah," said Jed. "Lock it up tight, then. I don't want anyone messin' with our stuff." Otis waved and walked away.

Jed shivered as the wind blew and he heard a low-pitched moan rising from the mouth of the cave, like some long dormant creature in pain had awakened. He turned toward the trailer and nearly tripped on the punky wooden steps. Before stepping inside, he tapped the sign next to the door proudly, which read *O’Donnell Construction*.

Empty beer cans and cigarette stubs left a stale odor in the trailer of a sports bar after Superbowl Sunday. Some dried-up half-eaten donuts lay discarded on the kitchen table. Down the hall toward the bunkroom, dirty clothes were strewn about the floor. Jed shook his head and grabbed his blueprint roll from the shelf along the wall. As a retired Army sergeant major, he couldn’t stand a mess, but he just shook his head, tired of babysitting grown men. He threw the stale donuts into the garbage can and wiped the table with a wet rag before unrolling the blueprints. While reviewing the plans, the violent sound of jackhammers outside was interspersed with yelling. He ignored the noises at first, because the boys always made a racket while they worked, but the noise persisted and raised his ire. He got up to look out the window. Scott Gurnsey was no longer on the backhoe. He stood on the edge of the trench by the ice cave facing toward Jed, yelling and waving his arms about wildly. Otis' head bobbed out of the trench briefly, only to disappear a moment later. Roger, who was kneeling over the edge of the trench watching his partners, suddenly jumped up and sprinted toward the trailer. Jed met him at the door.

"What the hell's goin' on?" Jed demanded.

"Otis found something in the trench," Roger panted. "Come on."

Jed reluctantly followed Roger over to the trench where the mist billowed out from the cave and down over the edge of the trench like steam from a geyser. Scott pointed down toward the opposite side, but the foggy mist moved in waves across the trench wall and obscured Jed's view. He squinted, but couldn't see anything, so he grabbed his bifocals out of his breast pocket. In between brief openings in the mist flow, he could only make out a small, brown object sticking out of the trench's side wall. The sound of the backhoe engine nearby was too loud for him to understand what Scott was yelling about.

"Roger!" Jed yelled pointblank into Roger's ear. "Get down in there and see what Scott's yappin' about." Roger obediently scurried along the edge of the trench to a spot where he could climb in. When he reached the opposite wall where Otis was, he began to wave his arms excitedly and point at the wall.

"Damn!" Jed swore. "Can't send a boy to do a man's work." He pulled up his pants and trudged along the edge until he was just above where Roger and Otis stood in the trench. Getting down on his hands and knees and peering over the edge he squinted and saw a glistening object about six inches long and three feet below, but he had trouble focusing with the mist fogging his glasses. He wiped his glasses with the back of his hand and bent his elbows to lean over the edge a little closer. "My God!" he gasped, as his eyes finally focused just before his glasses fell off. Jed's right hand slipped on the moist earth as he stabbed the air unsuccessfully to grab the glasses. Losing his balance, he nosedived into the trench as his face fell right into the cold, slimy, muddy human hand sticking out from the side wall. He grunted as he sat up at the bottom of the trench and wiped the mud off his face.

"You okay, boss?" Otis yelled in Jed's ear.

"Damn it, Otis! Damn! Tell Scott…go turn off the backhoe, you imbecile!"

Otis made hand signals to Scott to turn off the backhoe. A moment later, the backhoe engine wound down. The last gasp of the engine echoed across the lake, followed by deathly silence.

"What the hell?" Roger swore. "Let's get outta here." He turned to climb out of the trench and was followed by Otis.

"Get your asses back here!" Jed grabbed them by their pantlegs. He wasn't going to be frightened by a muddy hand. He'd seen much worse in Vietnam.

Sheepishly, Roger and Otis rejoined Jed. Scott returned from the backhoe and stood above them on the edge of the trench.

They all stared aghast at the hand as if it had just arrived from space. There was no doubt about it. It was human…and it appeared to be attached to a body.

"Let's get this poor sucker out of here," Jed said.

To avoid damaging the body, they used pickaxes and other hand tools like archeologists to carefully clear away the frozen shards of earth and patches of ice. After working non-stop for at least an hour, they were able to uncover the entire body. Its gray-colored skin was still intact and smeared with mud and ice shards. Surprisingly intact clothing was present, but tore away as they carefully extracted the stiff, frozen corpse from its tomb of ice and mud.

"Well…son-of-a-bitch!" said Jed. "Get the sheriff over here right quick."

2

Norm Phinney sat down at his desk to enjoy his morning coffee while reviewing laboratory results in the pathology office at the county hospital in Elizabethtown, New York. As he settled into his chair and savored his first sip, his aching knee joints reminded him that his fifty-year-old body was starting to feel its age. He scratched an itch on his cue ball-shaped head just as his desk phone rang. His triple-X-sized gut got in the way of him reaching to the other side of his desk for the phone, so he stood up and leaned forward to grab it.

"Norm," Sheriff Dave Egglegfield's voice came in clearly on the line, "a group of construction workers found something very curious out near Glacier Lake about an hour ago. I'll be bringing a body over to you shortly."

"I can hardly wait," Norm said sarcastically.

"I think you'll find it fascinating," Dave said. He then described in more detail exactly how and where the body was found. "And Norm…keep this under wraps for now, so we can avoid any public curiosity until we know what we're dealing with."

An hour later, Norm left his office for the loading dock in the back of the hospital to await the sheriff's arrival. A few minutes later, Sheriff Egglefield pulled up his van, got out, and gave Norm a nod. He opened the back of the van, revealing a white plastic sheet secured with rope and covering the outline of a body. Norm donned some gloves and rolled over a gurney that he'd wheeled up from the morgue. He helped Egglefield lift the body onto the gurney.

"He's pretty light," Egglefield said.

"Yeah," Norm said. "I'm surprised. Let's get him downstairs."

They wheeled the gurney into the freight elevator and down to the basement then pushed it through the dark, narrow hallways to the morgue. Once inside, they hoisted the body onto the dissecting table in the center of the room.

"So," Egglefield said, proudly, "check this out." He untied the rope, pulled off the plastic sheet and dropped it to the floor.

"Wow!" said Norm, giving the corpse a quick visual survey. "He's pretty shriveled up. Let me clean him up." Norm picked up a hose and gently sprayed the residual mud off the body, revealing cold, gray skin that looked like an old salami left in the fridge too long. "This is definitely one for the town history books, Sheriff. I've never seen anything like it. Kind of looks like a mummy."

"Yeah, I thought so, too. We've set up a perimeter around the location where he was found to see if we find any more bodies or evidence of foul play. I just want to make sure this isn't some unsolved murder case that I didn't know needed solving in the first place. So, if you can do anything to determine whether his death was natural or not, that would be helpful."

"Sure thing, Dave. From the looks of him, he's been frozen a long time, but I'll do what I can. I assume you'll be reviewing old records of missing persons?" Norm could feel his pulse quickening in anticipation of getting to work. This was truly something he hadn't seen before.

"Yeah. Standard protocol. Well, thanks," Egglefield said. "I'm heading back out to the site, so see you around."

Once the sheriff left, Norm was anxious to get started. He first walked around the dissection table, looking for any obvious abnormalities. Then he hastily set up everything he needed to do an autopsy. Since his diener who usually helped him was out of town, he'd have to do this one alone. He put on a lab coat, changed out his latex gloves, lined up his instruments, sample collectors, notebook, and camera. After taking a host of pictures and writing up a general description of the body, where it was found, and other basic information the sheriff had shared with him over the phone, he put down his pen and turned on his Dictaphone, so he could work hands free.

Norm proceeded with the first incision of any autopsy: a central "Y" cut to expose the chest and abdominal organs - something he'd done a thousand times, with careful, skilled hands. Norm held his scalpel and began with a cut at each shoulder in turn on a 30-degree angle slightly downward toward the breastbone in the center. Next, he proceeded straight down the middle of the chest and abdomen to the pubic bone. The tissue was still frozen and stiff, making it more difficult than usual to cut through. He had to use the weight of his body to lean in over the table to cut the tissue with his right hand, while balancing himself with the left hand against the corpse. As he was cutting down the skin over the breastbone the scalpel became stuck. He pulled down harder putting as much weight as he could behind it and suddenly, the tissue gave way. The scalpel tore through the remaining cadaver flesh and sliced clean through the glove on his left hand, deep into the side of his pinky.

"Shit!" he swore, as he dropped the scalpel, which clattered onto the floor. "Damn! Damn!"

Dazed and shocked by the stupidity of what he'd done, Norm clutched his wounded hand stood back from the corpse and nearly slipped on the floor, but he caught himself on a nearby desk. "Stupid idiot," he yelled. "Why didn't I wear my chain mail glove? Why didn't I wait until the stiff had thawed?"

When he recovered from the shock, Norm tore off his gloves and threw them into the trash, then examined the wound. The scalpel had sliced off a piece of tissue about a half inch wide and left a piece of flesh still hanging by a small stalk. He winced as he tore off the residual piece of tissue. Blood welled up at the base of the wound and trickled down his wrist. He rushed over to the sink and opened his first aid kit. He removed an antiseptic surgical scrub brushed and scrubbed his wounded finger raw.

3

Dr. Bill Denton was in the middle of an uneventful Friday family medicine clinic. He glanced at the day's schedule to see how the afternoon looked before standing up from the small desk in the exam room for a stretch. Outside his window he saw billowing clouds that left patches of shadows across the green valley, where lazy cows rested in the blossoming shade of maple trees. The scents of cow manure and mown grass wafted in through the window with the breeze. The scenery was quite a change from the view outside his office in Washington, DC, where the daily traffic flow, bustling pedestrians, and cacophony of horns and engines announced the progression of the day.

Bill glanced at the calendar, thinking about how long he'd already been back in Elizabethtown, a small hamlet in the middle of the Adirondack mountains where he grew up. He couldn't believe it had already been two months. His father, Alfred, asked Bill to return home to help run his medical practice while Alfred recovered from a mild stroke. What had begun as a good deed now gnawed at Bill like a toothache. Despite his desire to help his dad out in a pinch, one too many cases of routine hypertension, ear infections, and sore throats since his return challenged his interest in the daily grind of small-town medicine.

Bill stood nearly six feet tall, with a lean, muscular build, maintained by his rigorous daily workouts. He kept his hair cut above his collar and ears - a style he'd gotten used to during his ten years as an Army doctor. He still moved effortlessly with a quiet strength, his good physical condition making him look years younger than his mid-forties.

Bill massaged the base of his stiff neck, caused by leaning over his computer and patient charts too long, before returning to the desk. The description accompanying the next chart seemed routine: a six-year-old boy with a slight fever and vital signs otherwise normal. *Chief Complaint: rash.*

"Rosemary," Bill spoke into the intercom to reach his nurse, while reading the name on the chart, "please send Tommy in."

Angela Johnson and her son, Tommy, entered the room a moment later. Angela's smooth, round face and pageboy haircut made her look young enough to pass for a high schooler, but Bill estimated she was probably in her mid-twenties. Her slender body barely filled out her gray slacks and white cotton sweater. Bill recognized her as the much younger kid sister of one of his grade school friends.

Tommy fidgeted nervously, picking at his brown corduroy pants. Despite his slightly flushed face and unkempt brown hair, Bill quickly assessed from Tommy's alert demeanor that he was not severely ill. Even before Angela began to speak, Bill had observed the pattern and characteristics of a red, spotted rash on Tommy's face and arms as his mother helped the boy onto the exam table.

"Doctor," Angela began, "Tommy's been sick for about two days with a runny nose. Then last night, when I put him into the bath, I found these spots all over his chest."

"Any fever?" Bill leaned forward and began to write in the chart. He re-read Tommy's vital signs, taken by Rosemary, noting an oral temperature of 100.1 degrees.

"I think so, but I didn't have a thermometer…he just felt hot."

Bill then ran through a battery of questions: "Any diarrhea? Vomiting? Abdominal pain? Sore throat? Headache? Neck stiffness? Ill contacts? Current medicines? Allergies? Medical problems?" All Angela's responses were "No."

Bill put his pen down and rolled his stool toward Tommy.

"Well sport," Bill said, "you don't look very happy. How are you feeling?"

"Okay, I guess," Tommy responded, looking down at

his hands.

“Do you like to play sports? Basketball? Baseball?” Bill asked.

“Sure, baseball, but I’m kind of tired.”

“I’m not surprised,” Bill said. “Are any of your friends in school sick?”

“Uhm. I don’t think so,” Tommy said.

“Can you lift up your shirt, pal?" Bill asked as he pulled on some exam gloves.

Tommy pulled up his shirt, revealing many skin lesions, which Bill studied intently. He knew the diagnosis in seconds.

"See his rash?" Bill asked Angela. "Notice the difference in the lesions? Some are flat red spots, almost like a blood blister. Some look like pimples, with a little pus in them, and others have a dry scab.” Bill pointed out each type of lesion to Angela, touching them in turn on Tommy’s chest. “Plus,” Bill rolled the stool back to get a more complete view, “Tommy has more of them on his chest and back than on his face and arms.” Bill rolled forward again and pulled up Tommy’s pant legs. “Similarly, he has fewer on his legs. All of this is typical of chickenpox. In fact, he’s got a case right out of the textbook. Tommy, you’ve got chickenpox.”

"Chicken pops?" Tommy asked.

"Are you kidding me?” Angela asked. “That’s just great!” She threw up her arms.

“What’s the matter?” Bill asked, puzzled.

Angela folded her arms tightly across her chest and an expression of disgust crossed her face. “I told my mother he should get the shot, but *no.* She said ‘Don’t mess with nature. I’ve had it, you’ve had it. Let him get chickenpox.’”

Bill frowned. “There’s no doubt that a grandmother’s intuition has its place,” he said, “but even though chickenpox is generally benign for children Tommy’s age, it can have some serious consequences.” Bill paused to let that sink in. “But fortunately, those are rare. The new vaccine has proven to be very effective." Bill turned to Tommy, who eyed him nervously when he mentioned vaccines.

"Am I gonna get a shot?" Tommy asked, wincing.

"No. Don't worry pal. No shots today."

Tommy's expression relaxed. Bill helped Tommy pull his shirt back down. "Thank you, sport." Bill removed his exam gloves and tossed them into the garbage can before he washed his hands. Tommy grinned, revealing multiple missing teeth, when Bill handed him a lollipop.

"I thought that chickenpox was wiped out," said Angela. Bill leaned back against his desk wondering whether to launch into a discussion, but Tommy was the last patient of the morning, and he couldn't resist the opportunity to teach. "That's an interesting thought. The vaccine was licensed in 1995, so chickenpox cases have plummeted since we began using it. But it's only been two years, so we're not free of it yet. Hopefully we can get enough kids vaccinated, so that can be a reality some day. It even protects the few who aren't vaccinated."

"I'm not sure I follow you..."

Bill thought about an effective way to illustrate his point. "Think of it like this: if all of Tommy's friends get the chickenpox shot, his friends are protected, so the chance that Tommy will play with someone who has the chickenpox drops a lot. His friends act like an invisible shield to keep the disease away from Tommy, even if he doesn't get vaccinated. We call that 'herd immunity.' A person is protected from a disease by the immunity of the 'herd.'"

"I'm still not sure I get it."

"Well, try and think about it this way. It's kind of like in football the offensive linemen surround and protect the quarterback so he can throw the ball. Tommy's friends who are vaccinated are like the linemen."

"Ha," said Angela, "now I get it. Pretty cool. Maybe you could convince my mom about that. She's never even had a flu shot."

"Oh, I know," Bill said, "but I've dealt with a few stubborn patients before, including your mother. I am sure I'll have the opportunity to discuss her concerns the next time I see her."

"Maybe you could pretend to check out a book at the library," Angela suggested, "and accidentally run into her there."

"Maybe I will. I didn't realize she was still working there. If I don't see her there, she usually shows up when her prescriptions are running out – should be soon." Bill turned back to the desk and jotted down some final notes in the chart.

"Excuse me, Dr. Denton -" Rosemary's voice on the intercom startled Bill - "Dr. Phinney is on line 1 for you."

"Thanks, Rosemary. Can it wait?"

"I'm sorry, doctor, but he said it was important."

"Okay," Bill said, frowning. "Excuse me, Angela." Bill got up and left the room. He picked up the receiver in the hallway. "Hello?"

"Hey, Bill," Norm Phinney's voice boomed in his ear. "I hate to interrupt you during clinic -" Bill clenched his jaw and nodded silently in agreement - "but I've got something I *know* you'll want to see."

"Oh yeah?" Bill asked, unable to mask his annoyance. "What is it?"

"Awe, c'mon Bill," Norm implored. "You're always complaining about the mundane sniffles. I've got something incredible here – brought in by the sheriff this morning. I've never seen anything like it."

"Sure, Norm," Bill said skeptically. "You want me to come down to that dungeon?"

"What better place to commune with the dead?"

"Okay," Bill said, relenting. "I'm booked until the middle of the afternoon. Can it wait until I finish clinic?"

"Hmm, okay." Norm's voice betrayed his disappointment. "I guess this stiff's not going anywhere fast. I'll be waiting."

“Great. See you later.” Bill hung up the phone and re-entered the exam room. “Sorry for that interruption, Angela. Let’s make a plan for Tommy.” To Tommy’s delight, Bill prescribed several days off from school and a pile of good books and videos. “In a couple days, all his bumps should scab over, and he’ll no longer be contagious. Then he can return to school.”

“Okay, anything else, Doctor?" Angela asked.

Bill gave her a handout on measures to prevent Tommy from scratching his rash. “Say hi to your brother for me - haven’t seen him in ages. And don’t worry. I’ll track down your mother. I’m sure there’s some nasty medicine I can prescribe,” Bill said with a wink.

“Good idea. Thank you, Doctor.”

Bill patted Tommy on the head and said, "See you later, sport." Tommy grinned, his lips already stained purple from the lollipop.

After the Johnsons left, Bill washed his hands again before grabbing a sandwich from the refrigerator in the break room. He walked out to the reception room where Rosemary was busy annotating Tommy’s chart. She bore some resemblance to her brother, Henry O’Donnell, the town mayor. They both had fairly large frames. Her buxom figure comfortably filled out her starched white blouse and skirt. Her freckled cheeks had a perpetual pink hue, and her nose was upturned and sharp. Bill suspected she’d had some surgery on her nose, since he didn’t remember her having such a refined, pointed nose as a child. She kept her long reddish-brown hair tied up in a bun and had some light brown hair on her upper lip, which she attempted to hide with bleaching. Rosemary had been on the job a mere four months, but unfortunately she didn’t display the same skill or dedication as his father’s long-time nurse, who had retired just before his father’s stroke.

“Rosemary, why didn’t you put Tommy in the isolation room?”

“I’m sorry, Doctor,” Rosemary looked up from the

chart and blushed. "I didn't realize he had chickenpox until I read your note. When Angela brought him in, she just said he had a rash."

"Well, you need to be more careful," Bill scolded. "Any child with a rash should go straight into the isolation room. The last thing we need is a chickenpox outbreak." He withheld the urge to reprimand her more severely. "I guess we're fortunate on one account – he's the last patient of the morning. We should be able to air out the office before the afternoon patients arrive." Bill walked over to the window and lifted it. "Now that we've seen one case, I won't be surprised if we get some more. Can you wipe down the door handles and other surfaces with a disinfectant?"

Rosemary lifted her gaze. "Sure. I'll be on the lookout. We haven't seen much chickenpox here lately — seems like I used to see it all the time in nursing school."

"You're right," Bill said. He sat down next to the reception desk and pulled out his sandwich. "Maybe someday it'll be like measles."

"What do you mean?" Rosemary asked.

"You know, measles is so rare now, I only saw a few cases during my training, although we get periodic resurgences. I might not even recognize a case if one walked in today. Maybe someday it'll be the same for chickenpox. The older generation of docs treated all *kinds* of vaccine-preventable stuff that I've rarely, if ever, seen – you know, diphtheria, polio, and measles. Each generation sees fewer of the 'old' diseases."

"Oh, speaking of different generations," Rosemary said, reaching over to her in-box, "your father had a neighbor drive him into town. He dropped this off for you." She handed Bill a small white envelope.

"Great," Bill said sarcastically, reluctantly taking the envelope. "I wonder what advice he has today."

"Come on," Rosemary said with a grin, "go easy on your old man. Don't you think he just misses work?"

"I suppose so," Bill replied, as he shoved the envelope into his pocket without opening it.

"Do you think he'll be coming back to work soon?" Rosemary asked.

"Hard to say. He's made great progress since the stroke," Bill said in between bites of his sandwich, "so I don't see why not. It would probably do him good."

"Are you ready to leave town? I know that if I had the opportunity, I wouldn't hesitate to leave this place."

"Oh, really?" Bill asked. "I didn't realize you felt that way."

"Yeah, it's just kind of suffocating, with my brother being the mayor, and everyone knows everyone else's business. It would be nice to start over somewhere else."

Bill thought for a moment before responding. "I can understand that. For me, the change of scenery has been a nice break, but I really need to get back to my *real* job in the city. My boss won't give me much more time away."

"The patients will be sorry to see you go. After all, if something happened to your dad, all this town would have is that old geezer in Keene Valley or Dr. Tightwad."

"Who? Phinney?"

"Who else?" Rosemary rolled her eyes. "Your dad complains about him always trying to pinch pennies when it comes to patient care. It's probably better that he spends most of his time in the lab or the morgue. Most people would rather have you or your dad – better yet, you *and* your dad."

"I don't think that'll ever happen, but thanks for the compliment. Go easy on Phinney," Bill said. "He tries hard, even though he always seems to have some kind of get-rich-quick scheme up his sleeves." Bill finished his sandwich and got up. "I'm going to review some charts before the next patients show up. See you after your lunch break."

"Thank you, Doctor. Oh, by the way. What *did* Dr. Tightwad have that was so important?"

"Oh, thanks for reminding me…something about a

body the sheriff brought in…something he'd never seen before. Norm even piqued my interest this time. I'll head over to the morgue when clinic's over."

Rosemary shook her head. "Hmm. I'm sure it's *real* interesting," she said with a smirk. "Let me know what happens, though."

4

When clinic ended, Bill made the five-minute drive over to the hospital. One thing he really appreciated in Elizabethtown was the close proximity of everything and the minimal traffic. The center of town had only a single flashing red light. On the short drive, Bill passed the local grocery store, bank, hardware store, pharmacy, and multiple red-brick county government offices. He parked behind the hospital, a cream-colored single-story structure with a central building serving as the inpatient ward, one wing on the right as the emergency room, and the opposite wing as a nursing home facility. He walked through brightly lit hallways on the main floor and then descended the stairs to the basement. Down there the mood of the building took on a decidedly gloomy feeling as he navigated the darker maze of narrow hallways. The limited incandescent bulbs at 30-foot intervals in the ceiling left dark shadows lurking behind discarded, dust-covered equipment. The faded white stone walls dated back to busier days when the Adirondacks were a playground for the New York City upper crust and a sanctuary for tuberculosis victims. The hallway made him think of a tunnel of death, because any patients who didn't exit the building alive upstairs earned a one-way ticket through this tunnel to the basement morgue.

Bill's knocks on the heavy metal morgue door echoed down the lonely hallway. He squinted momentarily as the door squeaked open to reveal the brightly lit morgue, made more so as it reflected off Norm Phinney's shiny bald pate and tattered white lab coat.

"Bill! Glad you made it." Norm's round face broke into a broad grin. "Welcome to my chambers," he said with a laugh.

Norm was about five years younger than Bill and was shorter and pudgier, with a long brown mustache that consumed his upper lip. Both of them had grown up in town. Bill had followed Norm's career through their periodic contact over the years whenever Bill came to town to see his father. Norm was certified in family medicine, but he later switched to pathology. He had worked out an agreement with Bill's dad several years ago where they shared night call and management of the local 10-bed hospital and served as consultants at the adjacent nursing home. Norm ran the laboratory and morgue, which both served the surrounding regions as a referral center, while Bill's dad supervised the emergency room and inpatient ward. They hired a couple other contract docs from neighboring towns to help them cover the ER. The inpatient hospital usually didn't get a lot of business and Norm didn't see patients too often, so today, he wore his usual casual garb of shorts and a tee shirt under the open lab coat.

"It's cold and creepy down here," Bill said. "How can you stand to work in these catacombs?"

"Aw, c'mon Bill," Norm said, rubbing his bald head, "can't you think up something new? You know those hallways ward off the evil spirits and the riff raff so I can pursue my work without interruptions. Want some coffee?" He reached for a coffee mug on his gunmetal gray desk.

"No thanks," Bill replied, sitting down on a wooden stool. "The smell of formaldehyde in here brings back unpleasant memories of gross anatomy lab in medical school. My fellow anatomy partners used to eat during mini breaks while we were dissecting our cadaver, but my stomach couldn't handle it then and I still can't eat anything near it."

"Never bothered me." Norm belched before taking a long swig of his coffee. "My hands retain that glorious formaldehyde aroma for days." He sniffed his hands. "Hmm. What's that line from *Apocalypse Now*? I love the smell of formaldehyde in the morning?" He laughed at his joke.

"I still prefer living, breathing patients," Bill said.

"That's your mistake. My dead ones never complain.

And they *never* call me in the middle of the night." Norm grinned again while his mustache brushed over his teeth.

"I guess there is something to say for that," Bill said.

The morgue was a little better organized than the hallway. Four stainless steel refrigerator doors lined one wall, each with a large, hinged handle. The town didn't need such capacity for death anymore, except for the occasional multi-car accident. In the center of the room stood a shiny stainless steel dissecting table, which had rounded edges and looked like an elongated sink. The middle of the table had a gradual slope and funneled down to a drain, where a hose was attached and ran from the table down to a floor drain. A starched light green sheet covered the inner part of the table and Bill could make out the contour of a body underneath it. A long tan Formica laboratory bench ran along another wall, with a microscope situated in the middle and haphazard stacks of microscope slides around it. Three microscope viewing heads branched off the main microscope, like a three-headed dragon, so that multiple people could view a slide simultaneously. Bill noticed an old microscope discarded in the corner – residual of one of Norm's prior entrepreneurial endeavors that had gone nowhere. Bill couldn't remember exactly what that innovation was supposed to be. Norm's numerous degrees covered the creamy yellow walls, and every other surface was littered with computer carcasses.

"Norm, what's with all these computers?"

"We can talk about that later," Norm said impatiently. "Let's take a look at my surprise."

"Seriously, Norm. What's the deal?"

"Okay, what's another minute? It's simple: I'm trying to capitalize on the digital revolution."

"How so?"

"Okay. Well, you know how much space it takes to store all my pathology slides." He gestured toward a bank of special pathology file cabinets along the wall. "What if we could scan all our pathology slides and store them digitally?

Wouldn't that be cool?"

"Sure, but I don't think we have the computing power to do that yet."

"You are correct. The key is the word *yet*. It's coming my friend, maybe it'll take a couple years or a couple decades, but the pace is accelerating. So, all these computers are helping me build computing power to try and do this on a small scale. If I could patent a proof of concept, it could be worth millions."

"That would be pretty cool, I guess. So, good luck with it."

Norm frowned. "You don't sound convinced. You may not know, but I did computer programming in college, before I went to medical school."

"I think you may have told me that before," Bill said. Now he was sorry he'd brought up the subject. "I don't get it, though. With that kind of background, what keeps you here? Shouldn't you be working for some large computer company in a big city?"

"Yeah, but I spent enough years in the big city rat race before moving back here," Norm said. "I like the autonomy I have here with the multiple 'hats' I wear. I'm like the king of the mountain. There's not enough business in the surrounding country to sustain two pathologists, so I don't have to worry about competition, but anything new and exciting comes my way. Your dad has enjoyed this same type of monopoly with his clinical practice. Maybe you should consider taking over for him permanently. How's good old Alfred doing, by the way?"

"Looks like he's about ready to start seeing patients again," Bill said. "Maybe I can skip town soon. Anyway, you called me about something urgent. Show me what you've got."

"Yeah, like I said, anything new around here comes to me. So, first a little background." Like Dr. Frankenstein discussing his creation, Norm's eyes lit up and his arms moved about wildly while he described how the body had been discovered at a construction site that morning. "The sheriff brought me this stiff all covered in mud this morning. I drove over to check out the site this afternoon. I couldn't believe it. This sucker was entombed in a block of ice. You remember the ice cave?"

"You mean at Glacier Lake? Up by the Ausable Club? That was my favorite spot for playing hooky, plus all the best hiking trails start there for the Adirondack high peaks."

"One and the same, except I'm not much of a hiker, and by the time I was in high school, the school principal had it all figured out. He would send the vice principal out there to round up the miscreants."

"Too bad. I think my generation got a reprieve from the new vice principal, but look, Norm, don't stall any longer." Bill gestured toward the green sheet on the dissecting table. "Let's see the body."

"You asked for it." Norm put his coffee mug down on the lab bench. He wore a sinister grin as he walked over to the dissecting table and grabbed the edge of the green sheet.

Bill noticed Norm wasn't wearing gloves, and he felt the urge to turn his head as Norm gave the sheet a violent yank, exposing the upper body down to the thighs. Bill's eyes itched slightly as though flecks of something landed on them from the sheet. He blinked them away as if imagined, then he walked quickly over to the dissecting table. "Oh my God!" Bill gasped, as he stared down at the cadaver.

Gray skin stretched taut over prominent ribs and joints, like a suit shrunken two sizes in the dryer. Beneath the skin, the muscles seemed as if they had withered away, leaving mere sticks for arms and legs. The shriveled face and prominent cheekbones, without any fat below the surface, matched the skull's contours like a famine victim. Hollow eye sockets missing the eyes, were sunken in deep black pits like two snake holes. Lips, thin and cracked, drew up tight and opened over the teeth in a mocking grin like someone with a facelift from hell. Disheveled sandy-colored straight hair sprouted like weeds from the skull and pubic area, and below the pelvic bone hung a shriveled penis about the size of a breakfast sausage. Small brown spots barely protruding from the skin surface covered parts of the face, arms, and upper legs, with some surrounded by darkly pigmented rings. Some of the gray fingernails appeared darker than others, as if stained with walnut dye. A jagged gaping wound snaked down the center of the chest, stretched open by the tight skin.

"Wow! Norm, this is incredible! He's perfectly pickled, like a mummy."

Norm moved to the other side of the dissecting table. "Frozen, not pickled…but yes. Definitely amazing, nonetheless."

"Man, I knew it was cold up by that cave," Bill said, "but I never imagined it could do something like this." Bill leaned against the dissecting table. "Have you ever been in that cave?"

"Only once – in high school - on a dare," Norm responded. "Froze my ass off and scared the piss out of me. It was dusk, and that cave makes this gloomy sound when the wind blows. It was packed with snow and ice…and that was in the middle of August!"

"Pretty creepy to think that he could have been buried there all those times when we were goofing off or making a play for the girls." Bill shivered at the thought.

"I'll say," said Norm.

"Why is he so emaciated?" Bill asked. "Like he's been in a concentration camp? He's a lot scrawnier than the cadavers we dissected in medical school."

"You know what happens when you leave ice cubes in the freezer too long?" Norm asked.

"I guess," Bill answered, trying to picture old ice cubes. "Do they shrink?"

"Exactly," Norm said. "The same thing happens with a frozen body. Water evaporates over time - a process called sublimation. Because this poor sucker looks so dried up, I suspect he's been buried at least 50 years, maybe even 100, for all I know. It's hard to believe he'd stay preserved so long, like he was naturally embalmed."

"Well," said Bill, "I guess it's not too different from those stories you hear about cadavers being unearthed from the permafrost in Alaska or Siberia. We just happen to have our own little spot of permafrost at Glacier Lake. What's this gash down his central chest? Did they slice him during the extraction?"

"I wish," said Norm, looking sheepish. "In my eagerness to work on him, I made the mistake of thinking I could start the autopsy before he thawed. I got the scalpel caught in the frozen tissue. Unfortunately, when it released, I jabbed my pinky." He held up his left hand, demonstrating a large gauze bandage taped over his pinky, which made his finger look like a hot dog in a bun.

"Ouch!" Bill flinched. "Is it deep? You need me to stitch it?"

"Nah, just a flesh wound. Sliced a chunk of skin off." Norm blushed. "Hurt my pride more than anything. I haven't gaffed myself like that since I was a medical student."

"I noticed you weren't wearing any gloves when you uncovered him. Don't you worry about catching something – even if he's dead? I mean you hear all these stories about the 1918 flu from the cadavers in Alaska."

"Normally I wear a chain mail glove – but my eagerness got the better of me and I completely forgot. Besides, what could he have after all these years?"

"I don't know," said Bill, "but I'd prefer not to find out the hard way. Probably more of a risk of getting infected with some soil bacteria or fungus left on the cadaver's skin. Hand me a pair of gloves." Norm pulled purple nitrile gloves out of a box on the wall and handed them to Bill. Bill pulled them on before leaning closer to examine the body. “These dark brown spots are interesting. They look more prominent than freckles.” He ran a gloved finger over the skin. “They’re still slightly raised. Some look and feel like deflated balloons.”

“Yeah – they’re hard to miss. It’s possible they were more elevated at one time, but with the desiccation of the body, they’ve probably flattened out. What do you think they could be?”

“Hmm.” Bill stood back from the table to get a better viewing perspective, and he pulled down the rest of the sheet, exposing the entire body. "It's really hard to say. If this guy weren’t such a prune, then I might be able to imagine what they looked like when he was alive. Without that, I’m left with only their distribution pattern – looks like he’s got more of them on his face, arms, and legs than on his trunk. It also looks like he also might’ve had bleeding under the skin causing dark halo around some lesions. The pattern is opposite that of chickenpox,” Bill said, remembering Tommy Johnson from his morning clinic. “Even then, since chickenpox is less common in adults, it’s also more deadly in them. Maybe he had a real severe case of it. It’s hard to imagine, though, someone who’s sick hiking out into the woods and croaking. I mean, it’s a couple miles from the Ausable Club to the lake, and even with the new dirt road, it’s not much shorter. You need to be in good physical condition. I haven’t ever heard of chickenpox causing bleeding, though. Have you?”

Norm shook his head.

“If you’re thinking this guy’s been frozen for over 50 years,” Bill said, “that means he was buried in the 1950’s or even earlier. Hygiene then may not have been optimal. His lesions could be related to any number of things. Maybe they’re louse or flea bites? Maybe he didn’t even die from a disease at all. Maybe he just wandered off the trail in the middle of winter and froze to death. How do you piece it together?”

Norm leaned against the dissecting table. "It's impossible to say whether exposure was the ultimate cause or a contributing factor in his death. You're right about the bleeding, though. See this?" He lifted the cadaver's left arm and pointed to one of the larger lesions. "I incised it and there's a pocket of dried blood below the skin, so those rings are definitely bruises. I sent off some of that blood to our referral lab in Saranac Lake, since they have the capacity for more sophisticated bacterial and viral testing. I'm not naïve, though. I doubt they'll get anything to grow, but maybe they'll find something by PCR. The other thing I might try to do is take a piece of his spleen. That's usually a good way to find pathogens."

"I agree," said Bill. "So, what could've done him in? He doesn't look more than about 40."

"Probably natural causes," said Norm, "as I haven't seen anything to steer me otherwise, but I won't know for sure until I can do a full autopsy. Even then, I doubt I'll ever get a definitive diagnosis. My hunch is that something ate him up from the inside before he froze – something that can cause a rash with bleeding – maybe meningococcemia."

Bill straightened up from the dissecting table. Meningococcemia was deadly all right – a disease that occurred when the bacteria *Neisseria meningitidis* got into the blood stream. It could certainly lead to rapid death and severe bruising, called purpura. Bill was glad he wore gloves, although he wondered whether his clothes might have gotten some cadaver juice on them. "I'll be curious to know what you find when you finish," he said as he tore off his gloves and threw them into a red trashcan marked *hazardous waste*. He then washed his hands. "I need to get going – see what Dad's up to - but I'm really glad you called me, Norm. This was definitely worth seeing."

"No problem-o," Norm said, smiling. "I'll ping you once I finish the autopsy."

Bill opened the morgue door. "Make sure you take

care of your finger, or maybe I'll amputate it."

Norm nodded sheepishly.

Bill shut the door and walked back through the cinder block hallway toward the exit. Norm's impression had been right for a change. Bill had seen his share of frostbitten homeless people or hypothermic suicide victims pulled out of the icy Potomac River in winter, but this was something completely different. As he stepped out of the building, he took a deep breath. The smell of burning firewood in the air was refreshing and washed away the residual stench of formaldehyde from his nostrils. Cobble Hill, a mountain that towered over the west side of town with a peak as round as a ball was now silhouetted against the evening sky by the setting sun. As he reached into his pocket for his car keys, Bill felt the envelope that Rosemary had given him earlier and pulled it out.

How many of these ridiculous notes had he received from his father in the past two months? Five? Six? Ten?

Bill:

I hope you're not ordering too many lab tests on my patients. You know many are poor and don't have insurance. They can't afford anything that's not absolutely necessary.

Dad

"That's *it*!" Bill said loudly as he crumpled up the note in disgust and whipped it into a nearby dumpster. "So much for doing a good deed." He yanked out his keys and hopped into his beat-up old Chevy. He jammed the accelerator to the floor during the five-mile drive to his father's small village. On the way, he rehearsed exactly what he planned to say.

The latest note was the signal. Bill had been practicing medicine for nearly two decades, and he had worked in Army hospitals and field environments and lately in bustling cities. Of course he didn't order unnecessary tests. When his father started dictating how Bill should run the practice, it was time to leave. At one point in his career, Bill had contemplated sharing the practice full-time with his father, but he knew he would always be considered the "little boy." The numerous notes he'd received this visit proved that their dynamic would never change, and Bill could never tolerate the inevitable micromanaging.

Bill whizzed past a small green sign with white letters proclaiming *New Russia, Population: 50.* He crossed over a bridge and drove up a small knoll. The tires screeched as he hit the brakes as he reached the top of the knoll before making the first right turn onto a gravel driveway. He then drove through a grove of towering white pine trees into a clearing, which was dominated by his father's two-story white shingled farmhouse. A covered porch surrounded the house on three sides. Paint peeled from the edge of the roof awning and grass had cropped up between the slate walkway slabs. The left side of the house glowed orange from the sun setting behind Bald Peak, the towering mountain on the horizon. Bill jumped out of his car and stepped briskly up the porch steps into the house.

His father would usually be making dinner by this time, but the kitchen was surprisingly quiet, dark, and empty.

"Dad?" Bill called out, but there was no answer.

Bill's footsteps echoed on the hardwood floors as he walked throughout the house, checking one empty room after another. He finally found his father in the den staring at the television with a vacant expression, leaning onto the right armrest of a gray wicker couch. Something about him seemed different.

Bill picked up the remote control and shut off the television. "Dad," he said, "we need to talk." There was no answer. The old man just stared ahead with a blank expression.

"Dad, what's wrong?" Bill bent down and grabbed his father's chin, turning his face upward. Alfred's lips drooped on the right side and drool ran from the corner of his mouth down his chin. With each blink, only his left eye closed. His lips shook and he grimaced while attempting to speak, but he could only blurt out "...n...n…numb..."

"Damn!" Bill swore. He ran into the kitchen to call for an ambulance.

5

May 5 (D+1)

The screen door slammed behind him as Bill stepped off the porch onto the dewy grass outside his father's house. He squinted until his eyes adjusted to the morning light as rays of sunlight peeked through the majestic pine trees towering over the front yard. The cool morning air felt refreshing on Bill's face as he caught the scent of honeysuckle. He strolled past rotting tree stumps on a moss-covered pathway through the forest toward the road.

The birds singing in the trees in celebration of the spring day and the beautiful surroundings did little to lighten Bill's mood, though, as he was preoccupied with the recent developments with his father. As he walked, he pulled out his cell phone and called his boss in Washington, D.C.

"Hi Bob," Bill said, "Sorry this is taking longer than I anticipated. We just had a new setback last night, so now I can't predict how much longer this is going to take."

"Bill," his boss's baritone voice resonated through the receiver, "you can't stay there forever. The new intern class starts in about two months. You're their favorite professor on the wards, so I need you back here soon."

"I appreciate the flattery, Bob, but with my dad's new stroke last night, I really can't leave right now. Just give me enough time to straighten out whatever I can here, and then I'll come back."

"Sorry about your dad, but can you give me something more definite? I need to figure out how to cover for your patients and teaching."

"Maybe two, three weeks?"

Bob sighed on the other end of the line. "Okay. So that we don't have to have this conversation again, I'll give you some *very* generous wiggle room – up to 6 more weeks.

That would still get you back in time for the interns' orientation, but that as all I can do. If you aren't back here by then, your job may be at risk. Some of the new guys in the department are starting to grumble about having to cover your patients. It's only a matter of time until one of them goes over my head to the Dean."

"I understand. Thanks, Bob. I'll be in touch. If it looks like it'll take more than 6 weeks, I'll call the Dean myself. I'll make it up to you."

"Be careful what you promise…"

Bill shut off his cell phone as he crossed the road to the New Russia Post Office. The small gray building stood alone next to the road, its weather-beaten white shingles dulled by the harsh Adirondack winters. Nettie Baker, the Postwoman, wore a brown housecoat and kept her short gray hair tucked under a green handkerchief. She sat in an Adirondack chair on the porch surrounded by a haze of smoke.

"Good morning, Nettie," Bill called as he approached.

"Morning. How are you, Doc?" Nettie asked, with a deep, hoarse voice.

"I've had better days." Bill grabbed her arm to help her up from the chair.

Nettie had been the Postwoman since Bill was a boy, and he knew her arthritic joints bothered her, even on this spring morning. Nettie took one long puff on her cigarette, savoring it as if it were her last breath, and then she opened the screen door, leaving a trail of smoke behind her. Bill instinctively held his breath as he followed her inside. The Post Office only had a single room about the size of a small kitchen. It was split down the middle by an open oak countertop and a bank of tarnished brass post-office boxes that rose to the ceiling. The familiar stench of stale cigarette smoke hung in the air and clung to the worn olive-colored chairs and brown carpet inside.

"You look upset," Nettie said as she walked behind

the counter. "Has Alfred been grumpy?"

"Unfortunately, I wish that were the case," Bill replied.

"Oh?" Nettie leaned forward over the counter and grabbed his hand with her bony fingers. Blue snake-like veins coursed across the backs of her hands and between her knobby knuckles.

"Dad's worse," Bill said. "He had another stroke last night."

Nettie gasped and put her hand to her mouth, then she grabbed Bill's hand so tight he could feel the blood draining from his fingertips.

"Yeah," Bill said, releasing his hand from Nettie's grasp. "It's horrible. I spent a good part of the night with him at Saranac Hospital. He'll probably be there for another day or so." Bill sighed. He ran his hand through his hair and kicked his foot against a hole in the carpet. "This second stroke's more debilitating than the one he had in March. In fact, I can't predict what kind of function he'll end up with. It's pretty bad."

"I'm so sorry, Bill." Nettie walked out from behind the counter and gave him a tight hug.

"I'm not sure how he's going to deal with this," Bill said. "He'll go crazy if he can't work. You know how much he loves his patients and independence."

"I know." Nettie's distraught eyes glistened with tears as she sat down in a threadbare chair next to the window. She pulled a handkerchief out of her pocket and blew her nose. "And what are we going to do without him?" She shook her head and frowned, wrinkling up her prune face. "Your dad and I have been in this one-horse town longer than anyone. I don't know what to say. Is there anything *I* can do?"

"Well, I *was* hoping you could help me out," Bill said as he sat down next to her.

"Anything, Doc." She patted his knee with her bony hands.

"I remember several years ago you had to get a live-in nurse for your father. You seemed pleased with the assistance. Where did you find her? I need to find someone for Dad."

"Wouldn't he be better off in some kind of care home?" Nettie asked. "I thought you weren't planning on hanging around."

"I'm not," Bill said, "but I need at least a temporary set-up until I can find a quality long-term place for him…probably close to me in Washington."

"Of course," Nettie said. "The agency I used was very professional and does a lot of work with the state hospitals. I may even have the number somewhere around here." She got up and walked back behind the counter and rummaged through some files. "Ah, here it is." She returned and handed Bill a wrinkled slip of paper, then she sat down again. "They're over in Saranac. If you act fast, they'll visit him in the hospital before he gets discharged, and they'll want to evaluate the house, too, to see if any modifications are needed."

"This is great," said Bill, as he thumped the paper. "Thank you. I'll call them later this morning." Bill got up to leave.

"Is it okay if I tell others about Alfred's condition?" Nettie asked. "They might want to visit him in Saranac."

"Sure," Bill said. "Please do."

Bill wasn't surprised by Nettie's question. Nettie had a legendary interest in town gossip, but in the positive sense. With her position at the Post Office, neighbors freely shared details about their lives, but if something was fairly sensitive, she kept it to herself. However, if the news could be beneficial to spread, she willingly told everyone. Bill suspected all 50 townspeople in New Russia would know about his dad by the end of the day, and that was a good thing.

"Thanks. I'll spread the word. Oh, Bill, before you leave, I heard the sheriff found a dead body up at Glacier

Lake. Know anything about it?"

Bill suspected Nettie already knew more than he did. Nevertheless, he described what he had seen in the morgue but withheld some of the gory details.

Nettie leaned back in her chair and lit up another cigarette. A thin curl of smoke flowed from the tip, which gradually unwound and widened into a band as it floated upward.

"When I heard about this yesterday," Nettie said, "I got to thinking. These Adirondack peaks are still pretty wild - seems like every couple years some poor soul gets lost hiking in the hills. It might take a couple years, but they generally turn up, rotted on some hillside. There's only one time I remember they didn't find 'em. I think I was a teen around then – shortly after World War II. Gosh, I can't believe it's been so long. There was this fella everyone was looking for."

"Boy, that really is a long time," said Bill, intrigued by Nettie's story. "I remember when old man Morris disappeared in the middle of winter when I was in high school. His grandchildren found his body in the woods the following summer. How can you remember something so long ago?"

"Oh, I'd forgotten about it completely…until I heard about that body, but it was a big deal when I was little. Yes sirree. Seemed like everyone was after this guy."

"After him?" Bill asked. "For what reason? Who was he?"

"Beats me. I told ya, I was just a teen. I forgot to ask my parents when I got older…some fella from far off…You'd ha' thought he'd killed somebody."

"Did he escape from Dannemora prison up north?"

"We've had our share of escaped convicts from there hiding out in the woods," Nettie said, "but no, I don't think so. He came from south of here, maybe New York City. Beyond that, I don't remember, but it was a big deal. My momma was real scared, and the sheriff told everyone to stay inside. That wasn't hard, because I remember we had a big ice storm around then. Even the Canadians were all riled up. Yeah, he must've done somethin' *real* bad."

"So, you're sure they never found him?"

"Not that I reckon," Nettie said. She took a long hit on her cigarette. Smoke puffed out of her mouth and nose as she spoke. "After about a month, the whole thing blew over. I think they figured he got lost somewhere between here and Canada or maybe left the country."

"That's an interesting story," Bill said. "I wonder if there's any record of it in the old newspapers."

"Maybe in the library," Nettie suggested.

"I'll try and remember to ask the sheriff if he's ever heard about it, but it's before his time, too," Bill said. He glanced at his watch. "Whoops! Nettie, I really need to get going. My clinic starts soon. Thanks for the help with the nursing service. See you tomorrow – have a good day." Bill waved as he left. He chuckled to himself as he hurried out of the post office and headed back toward the bank of pine trees across the road. He could always count on Nettie for some genuine, small-town yarns. An image of the shriveled cadaver briefly flashed into his mind. Could that man be the one Nettie remembered?

"Make sure to ask if you need anything, ya hear?" Nettie called after him.

Bill responded with a wave.

6

May 11 (D+7)

Norm Phinney awoke earlier than usual. A gnawing, throbbing pain from his left pinkie finger had kept him up most of the night. He got out of bed and splashed water on his face, but even the touch of water on the wound sent sharp pains up his arm. He also felt a sharp pain under his left arm pit. He reached up there and felt an oval, rubbery, swollen, tender lymph node about an inch wide. He studied the wound on his left hand. It was covered with a rough, dark brown scab, but his finger had swollen to double its normal size, like a mozzarella stick, with beefy red tissue and pus oozing around scab. He stumbled like a drunk to the kitchen for breakfast, still wearing his pajamas. While munching on a bowl of cereal, he felt the sudden onset of a chilly sensation, then his arms and legs began to shake rhythmically while his teeth chattered uncontrollably and he sweated profusely. "Damn. I must have the flu," he thought and took his temperature: 103 degrees.

He gulped down as much water as he could, nearly spilling half of it on himself in the process, then he headed back to his bedroom and climbed into bed. Despite a mountain of covers, he continued to shiver, as he drifted off into oblivion.

7

May 18 (D+14)

Dr. Alfred Denton sat motionless in the easy chair by the bed while Laura Chen tidied up his room. Petite, with straight black shoulder-length hair and clipped bangs, Laura moved effortlessly around the room as she made the bed, swept the floor, and wiped down the side table and bookshelf. This was her first assignment as a live-in home health nurse, so she wanted to make a good impression. Dr. Bill Denton hired her within days of Alfred's second stroke. In the two weeks since then, Laura knew she'd made the right decision in taking the job.

She smiled at Alfred, but he didn't acknowledge her and continued to stare out the window. His poor food intake had begun to concern Laura. Unlike many of her previous stroke patients in the hospital, who had to be fed through feeding tubes, Alfred was fortunate to still have a gag reflex, so he could eat without choking, but his right-sided paralysis created a strange contrast between both sides of his face, giving him the appearance of a dramatic mask expressing happy and sad emotions simultaneously. His right arm and leg, partially limp from the stroke, hung down at his side, like dangling spaghetti strands. The worst effect of the stroke was on the part of his brain that was vital for communication. Patients with similar strokes, called a Broca's aphasia, understood what others said to them and could even formulate a response in their mind, but couldn't express words properly. Consequently, when Alfred spoke, the words were choppy and often incoherent. His expressions whenever he tried to communicate showed Laura how frustrated he was.

Alfred's right-sided weakness was not so severe that he couldn't care for many of his daily needs with assistance, but Laura still assisted him with physical therapy, bathing, medication administration, moving about the house, and preparing meals. A visiting speech therapist had also started working with him.

"Dr. Denton," she called. "I'm going to do a quick workout before I prepare dinner. Can I get you anything first?"

The old man's eyes met hers momentarily, and then he shook his head sullenly.

Laura walked down the hallway past a large African spear and shield and two scowling brightly colored wooden masks, before climbing the creaking wooden stairs to her room. Except for some of the African decorations, the house was the kind of place she had envisioned when she thought of the Adirondacks. Most rooms had stained knotty pine paneling and wide-planked maple hardwood floors covered with faded red and green throw-rugs. Tall, open ceilings downstairs displayed large, cracked beams that extended the length of each room. A huge stone fireplace dominated the living room.

Her bedroom reminded her of an old country inn. The age-darkened knotty pine walls displayed prints of Adirondack scenes: an old logging camp, a tuberculosis sanatorium in Saranac Lake, and an Adirondack lodge. Blue curtains with brown covered wagons adorned the windows, and a white down comforter blanketed her mahogany poster bed. Her window overlooked the gravel driveway, which was partially covered with pine needles.

Laura changed into a T-shirt and sweatpants and commenced her daily routine, first with ten minutes of stretching, followed by yoga. The long hallway upstairs served as a runway for her to practice tai chi, which she'd learned from her grandfather. As she took regular deep breaths and began slow, rhythmic movements, she reminisced about him. She could still smell the dried mushrooms, exotic roots, and other earthy fragrances in his herbal shop in Chinatown, which she used to explore as a child. After spending a year caring for her grandfather as he was dying of cancer, she decided to become a nurse.

Once warmed up, she engaged in a series of more vigorous boxing moves, followed by free weights. A close call with a mugging while in nursing school convinced her of the need to be physically fit for self-defense, and a determination not to be so vulnerable in the future.

After a quick shower, Laura felt energized as she skipped back down the stairs to make dinner. The kitchen stood in contrast to the rest of the quaint house, with sheetrock kitchen walls painted a dull yellow. Olive-colored 1970-era appliances, with years of caked up grease, were in desperate need of replacement. The kitchen could definitely use some work.

Laura was in the mood for Chinese stir-fry. She pulled some strips of chicken breast out of the refrigerator that she'd already marinated in soy sauce, garlic, ginger, cooking wine, and a pinch of sugar. Next, she methodically chopped broccoli, bell pepper, carrots, and an onion, one-by-one to the exact size for proper cooking. While she worked, she periodically gazed out of the large picture window toward two horses grazing in the neighbor's field. On the opposite side of the field, Bald Peak rose up from a dense evergreen forest, where its patchy white rounded top dominated the horizon. The sun, now casting a burnt orange glow, had moved behind the left side of the mountain.

Laura brought many of her own cooking utensils and spices, since the house was not well equipped for her style of cooking. She rinsed some rice and started the rice cooker. She then drizzled canola oil into a wok, followed by the marinated chicken strips, which sizzled as they hit the hot metal. She grabbed a metal spatula and began to sauté the meat. The kitchen filled with the aroma of searing garlic. When the chicken was well cooked, she set it aside in a bowl and replaced it with the chopped vegetables that steamed as they cooked.

She secretly hoped that Bill might show up in time for dinner. Although she enjoyed the freedom of the current work, she missed having someone to converse with during the day. The little contact they'd had thus far had been pleasant, even though Bill was understandably preoccupied with work and his father's illness. For a fleeting moment, she wondered how a good-looking guy his age wasn't already married, but she knew it was none of her business. Besides, it didn't really matter. She'd dated more than her share of doctors, and she really wasn't interested in complicating her life right now. This was a job – a good one, but it was temporary - until Bill could find a more permanent place for Alfred. Experience had taught her not to think otherwise.

Once the vegetables were done, Laura tossed the chicken back into the wok and voila, the meal was ready. She scooped rice onto two plates followed by the corresponding portion of chicken-vegetable stir-fry. She took one of the plates down the hall for Alfred.

8

At the end of his Friday clinic, Bill was in his office packing his briefcase when there was a pounding on the door. Without waiting for an answer, in walked Norm Phinney.

"I hate to bother you," Norm said quietly with a raspy voice, "but Rosemary said it was okay."

"No problem, Norm," Bill said, standing up to shake Norm's hand. He gestured toward a chair next to the desk. "Have a seat."

"Thanks. I'm a bit embarrassed coming here," Norm said, appearing surprisingly subdued and a bit pale.

"Don't be ridiculous, Norm. My door's always open. Is this a medical issue?"

"Yeah. I don't usually consult anyone about myself."

"You and me both. What's on your mind?"

"Remember, about two weeks ago I nicked myself with a scalpel?"

"Yes," said Bill, "you mean while cutting on that frozen corpse?"

"Right. Well, a couple days later, my left pinkie was sore as hell." Norm cradled his hand as if the finger still hurt. "I got the shakes and a high fever for about a week. Man, I was sick as a dog and couldn't even get out of bed; otherwise, I might have come to see you sooner."

"I wish you had," Bill said, frowning. "If you had gotten septic, we might not even be having this conversation. Let me see your finger." Norm hesitated before slowly extending his hand for Bill's examination. Bill assessed a rough, dark brown scab about the size of a dime at the base of Norm's pinkie, which had a ring of redness about a quarter inch wide. "How did it look before?"

"Much worse. My finger swelled up like a hot dog and my hand puffed up like a baseball mitt. The lesion turned into a big pocket of pus. It was so painful I couldn't even tie my shoe. I ended up taking some ciprofloxacin, because I had some left over and I didn't want to buy any more antibiotics. I've been in bed ever since."

"You probably had a Staphylococcal infection. Unfortunately, cipro's not that useful for Staph. If I had known you were that sick, I might have thrown your ass into the hospital." Bill yanked on a pair of gloves and ran his hand over the bumpy scab. There was still some swelling around the scab, but he didn't feel any soft, puffy areas where pus might be hiding. He turned Norm's hand around to view the lesion from several different angles. The color, shape, and texture of the lesion seemed vaguely familiar. He ran his hand up Norm's arm. There were no red streaks coming from the wound, but he did feel a dime-sized rubbery lymph node on the inside of Norm's arm, just above the elbow and a quarter sized, mobile lymph node in his armpit. Norm winced when Bill palpated those areas. "It looks like it's healing, but I wish I could've seen it before. You do still have some tender, swollen lymph nodes."

"Yeah, I know. They were definitely a lot bigger a couple days ago. Sorry I didn't come in sooner," Norm replied sheepishly.

"You know the old saying: 'a doctor who treats himself has a fool for both a doctor and a patient.'" Bill tore off his gloves and discarded them before washing his hands.

"Don't remind me. Do I need to do anything else? My fever and chills are gone."

Bill sat back for a moment and considered the options. "At this stage, I could take a culture, but to do that, I'd have to pick off the scab to get some fresh fluid." Norm cringed at that possibility. "Don't worry. Since it seems to be resolving on its own, I won't mess with a good thing. But because you still have some redness and the tender lymph nodes, I'd like to switch you to an antibiotic that's more effective against Staph. I'll write you a script for cephalexin."

"You have any free samples?"

"Sorry, no."

"Dr. Denton?" Rosemary appeared at the doorway. "Excuse me, but a Mrs. Whitman just called. Her six-year-old boy is sick with a temperature of 103. Should I tell her that you're closed for the day? I suppose she could take him to Keene Valley's all-night clinic."

"What?" Bill asked. "Absolutely not! That's a good 20 miles away. Tell her to bring him in immediately." Rosemary nodded with a frown and disappeared from the doorway.

Norm let out a chuckle. "Seems like the train wrecks always show up on Friday afternoon."

"That's definitely true, but it's not funny," Bill said, annoyed by Norm's and Rosemary's callous attitudes. Bill lowered his voice and closed the door. "I wonder about Rosemary's compassion sometimes. She occasionally forgets that patient care doesn't go just from 9 to 5."

Norm stood up. "I haven't, and that's why I don't do it much anymore. I'm not the most dedicated doc on the planet, and I'm humble enough to admit it, but I'm glad that there are still guys like you around, Bill. I'll get out of your way, so you can take care of business."

"Here – Bill scribbled a script – "I prescribed you seven days of antibiotics."

"Thanks," Norm said as he took the script. "I'll let you know if anything changes. Good luck with the boy and call me if you have any urgent lab requests. That *is* something I can help with." Norm winked, showing a bit of his usual jovial personality again, and then left.

A few minutes later, Rosemary came in with Jeremy Whitman and his mother. The two of them helped the wiry, red-haired Jeremy up onto the exam table, where he promptly curled up and closed his eyes. Mrs. Whitman and Rosemary rolled stools up next to the other side of the exam table.

Bill didn't recognize either of the Whitmans. "Are you new to these parts?"

"Yes, doctor," Mrs. Whitman responded. "We've only been here for about six months."

"Well, I'm glad to meet you, although I wish it could be under happier circumstances. Jeremy doesn't look like he's feeling too well, but hopefully we can figure out why." During his years of experience, Bill learned the importance of visual observation of a patient -- how they act, their skin tone, their breathing pattern. He knew immediately that Jeremy was very ill. After pulling on a pair of gloves, Bill began to examine him closely.

"What are his vital signs?" he asked without looking up.

"104 degrees, oral," Rosemary said. "Pulse – 140."

In addition to the fever and elevated pulse, Jeremy was breathing fast – probably around 25 breaths per minute, and his breaths were labored. It was not uncommon for the pulse and the breathing rate to increase as the fever rose, but both were faster than he would have expected from just the fever. Jeremy's skin was flushed, warm, and dry, indicating he might be a bit dehydrated. Even when children are ill, they can be distracted with things like candy and toys, but when Bill brought those out and tried to humor Jeremy, he showed no interest.

"How long has he been like this?" Bill asked.

"He started acting tired two days ago," Mrs. Whitman said. "I had to pick him up early from school. He's been in bed ever since. He won't eat or even watch TV. I figured he might just have the flu, but I got *real* worried when I saw those bumps on his face."

Bill assessed all the information he heard and observed. Not wanting to eat was another sign of a sick child, and it was too late in the year for influenza. Numerous tiny bumps were scattered on Jeremy's face and appeared on first glance to be pimples. On closer inspection, they had dimples and some clear fluid in their centers. Bill ran his gloved index finger over them. They protruded slightly from the skin surface and rolled, firm, between his fingers, like BB pellets. He lifted Jeremy's shirt, revealing fewer scattered bumps on his chest and back.

"Did Jeremy get the chickenpox vaccine?"

"Yes, doctor. He's had all his shots. Do you think it's chickenpox?"

"I'm not sure," Bill said, surprised by her answer, because chickenpox was at the top of his list of possible diagnoses. He completed his examination by looking in Jeremy's mouth and ears, listening to his heart and lungs, and then feeling his abdomen. "He appears more ill than most kids I've seen with chickenpox, and the pattern of the rash is not quite typical."

"But if he's been vaccinated, how could he get chickenpox?" Mrs. Whitman asked.

"Good question. Not everyone who's vaccinated develops resistance to infection. Even with the best vaccines, people can still get a disease, especially if they have a large exposure."

"What if it isn't chickenpox?"

Bill sat down on his stool and thought for a moment. There were a couple other childhood rashes that could look similar early on, such as insect bites, poison ivy, scabies, a drug reaction, or even herpes, although the children usually don't appear so ill. "There are some other possibilities. Is anyone else sick at home?"

"My husband and daughter just left for a class trip to Washington, DC, but they've been fine, and I haven't had anything, either."

"What about other sick children?" Bill asked. "Any of his friends? Any insect or tick bites? Did he start any new medicines or supplements?"

"Not that I know of," Mrs. Whitman responded.

"We saw a case of chickenpox here recently, didn't we, Rosemary?" Bill asked. "About two weeks ago?"

"Yes," Rosemary said. "Tommy. In fact, he was the

same age."

"Oh wait," Mrs. Whitman said, excitedly, "do you mean Tommy Johnson?"

Bill nodded.

"I'd completely forgotten," Mrs. Whitman said, "but Jeremy played with Tommy about two weeks ago. His mother even *told* me he got chickenpox the day after they played. Sorry I forgot about that," she said quietly and lowered her eyes.

Bill smiled. "That's okay," he said. The pieces of the puzzle were starting to fit together. "Patients with chickenpox are most contagious just before the rash appears, and the incubation period would be about right, then," he said.

"What's that, Doctor?" Mrs. Whitman asked.

"Oh, sorry," Bill responded. "An incubation period is the amount of time it takes someone to get sick after they've been exposed to a disease. It's around two weeks for chickenpox. The timing would be perfect for him to be sick right now." Bill paused for a moment. Sweat glistened on Jeremy's back, which immediately soaked through his shirt when Bill pulled it back down. Bill still had some nagging concerns about how ill Jeremy appeared, despite the timing.

"Anyone in the family have herpes?"

"No." Mrs. Whitman responded with an air of disgust.

"Please don't take my question the wrong way," Bill explained. "Herpes is a common infection and can cause a generalized rash like this, especially during the first episode. Also, some kids can have more severe chickenpox if they have other illnesses, like AIDS or leukemia, which weaken their immune systems. I don't think Jeremy has anything like that, but I'm concerned enough that I want to watch him in the hospital for a couple days. I'll give him medicine through his veins that works against both chickenpox and herpes."

Mrs. Whitman's face blanched at this notion. "Can I stay with him?"

"Of course. Before we move him there, though, I'd

like to take a sample from one of his bumps for testing."

Bill left the exam room and walked down the hall to a small lab that his father kept for routine procedures like drawing blood and taking throat cultures. Although he'd used items in the refrigerator before, he wasn't completely familiar with everything his father kept on hand. He hoped he would find some viral culture media. Inside the freezer, he noticed several vials of vaccines and a small vial off to the side filled with white powder. The label read: *Dryvax - Wyeth labs.* He wasn't familiar with it, and put it back, making a mental note to ask Rosemary about it later. The door of the freezer held a vial with the familiar pink fluid he was looking for. He warmed the vial in his hands as he returned to the exam room, grabbing a glass microscope slide on the way.

"Rosemary," Bill said, looking around the room, "do we have any rayon swabs?"

"Not that I know of, doctor," Rosemary said.

"Okay, I'll use cotton then. You may feel a bit of a pinch, Jeremy, but it'll be over before you know it." Jeremy didn't seem to care. Mrs. Whitman held the boy's hand and rubbed his forehead.

"What do you need, Doctor?" Rosemary asked.

"Let's see," said Bill. "An alcohol wipe, a sterile scalpel blade, a cotton swab, and a bandage.

Rosemary laid all the items on a portable table. Bill then wiped one of the larger lesions on Jeremy's chest with the alcohol pad. Jeremy winced when Bill nicked the lesion with the scalpel. Clear fluid oozed out. Bill rotated the cotton end of the swab on the base of the lesion to gather cells and fluid and placed the swab tip into the vial. He broke off the stem and screwed the vial shut. "I'll send this to a lab over in Saranac Lake," Bill said. "They have better capabilities than we have here locally. They'll incubate it for several days, sometimes weeks, to see if a virus grows." He dropped the vial into a plastic bag and handed it to Rosemary, who was making a label for it. "Okay, Jeremy, this time I'm just going to scrape the bump. It will still hurt, but not as much. Is that okay?" Jeremy nodded slowly. Bill scraped the scalpel blade across the surface of the lesion some of the fluid the scalpel picked up on a glass microscope slide. He set the slide next to the sink in the exam room. "There. All done, sport." Bill felt relieved that Jeremy's lips turned up in a brief half-smile.

Rosemary opened the bandage and covered the lesion, then she left momentarily and returned with a wheelchair. Mrs. Whitman and Rosemary helped move Jeremy onto the wheelchair. Bill and Rosemary removed their gloves and washed their hands. Bill followed the three of them outside to the car. "I'll call over to the hospital," Bill said, "so someone will meet you at the entrance. I'll drop by in a little while to check on him. If you have any problems, have the nurse on the floor page me."

"Thank you doctor," Mrs. Whitman said.

When the Whitmans had driven off, Rosemary reluctantly agreed to drop off the viral culture sample at the local hospital lab on her way home, so that Norman could ship it to the more sophisticated lab in Saranac Lake. Bill phoned the hospital to let them know about the admission, then he carried the glass slide to his father's lab. The lab was rudimentary, but fairly well stocked with an assortment of blood tubes, syringes, needles, cotton swabs and pads. Several clear bottles filled with colored stains stood next to the sink. He held the slide with a pair of tweezers while waving a lit match under it to dry and bind the lesion scrapings onto the slide. Then he reached for a bottle with a purple solution in it, labeled *Gram's Stain.* He used a stopwatch to ensure the stain stayed on the slide for the proper amount of time before pouring on a brown iodine fixer solution. Again, after awaiting the appointed time, he next used alcohol to remove some of the Gram's stain to allow for a pink counter-staining solution. When the staining process was completed, he air-dried the slide and evaluated it under the microscope. If bacteria caused Jeremy's rash, they would appear as tiny purple or pink spheres or rods under the scope. Instead, sheets of much larger white blood cells filled his view. They appeared like fried eggs, only the egg whites were stained pink and the yolks purple. Bill saw no bacteria, and most of the white blood cells visible were lymphocytes, something more commonly seen with an illness being caused by a virus, like varicella, the cause of chickenpox, than a bacteria. Unfortunately, viruses were just too tiny to be seen with a light microscope, so Bill would have to await the results of the viral culture from the Saranac Lake lab to be sure.

Back in his office Bill rubbed his forehead and contemplated how to treat Jeremy. Years ago, when he was in the Army, he'd cared for a young soldier who had died of varicella pneumonia. It was rare, but some individuals, especially those with immune compromise or pregnancy could become severely ill. That soldier had been admitted to the hospital too late for any treatment to be beneficial. The same would not happen with Jeremy, he hoped.

Bill phoned the hospital again and dictated his orders to the floor nurse: an isolation room restricting access only to individuals who have had chickenpox or received the vaccine; intravenous fluids for Jeremy's dehydration; vital signs every two hours; numerous lab tests, including varicella and herpes antibody titers; and intravenous acyclovir, a drug to treat herpes viruses, 200 milligrams every 8 hours. Bill hoped it would help Jeremy turn the corner.

9

Laura sat at the kitchen table with an old textbook she'd found on the bookshelf in Alfred's study. Alfred was already resting in his room after dinner. Homemade pumpkin pie, spinach casserole, and venison steak, were piled on the kitchen counter or already stored in the fridge after being brought by Nettie and other well-meaning neighbors who had heard about Alfred's second stroke.

With the generosity of the neighbors, after tonight, Laura didn't have to worry about cooking for a couple days, so she had the opportunity to indulge in her passion for medical history. Her interest in history and folk remedies began with her grandfather but had been nurtured by her mother's interest in Chinese herbal medicine. She was delighted to find Alfred's home medical library replete with some exciting sounding titles like *Rats, Lice, and History*, *Anatomy of an Epidemic*, *The White Plague,* and *Inside the Hot Zone*. She resolved to take advantage of any free time to read as much as possible.

She looked outside, hoping to see how the evening calm had settled across the forest, but instead, the kitchen light caused her to see her own reflection in the kitchen window. Her reflection disturbed her, as she looked pale and ghostlike as a translucent figure.

She shuddered and took her eyes away from the window and looked down at the medical history book, opening the worn cover and turning the brittle yellowed pages, releasing a puff of dust in the process.

As a whippoorwill outside bid a haunting farewell to the day, Laura went back in time to learn about novel approaches to disease prevention and treatment before the discovery of antibiotics. She took out a pen and paper and scribbled notes as she read.

While she read about Ignaz Semmelweis' 1841

discovery that hand washing could prevent deaths from infection during childbirth, car lights shone through the window followed by the sound of a car door squeaking open and slamming shut. Laura glanced at her watch: 9:00. Her pulse picked up slightly as the kitchen door opened.

"Hi Laura," Bill said as he walked in carrying a load of books and files. "Wow, something smells good."

"Just a little stir fry. Have you eaten?"

"No, I'm starved. Sorry I'm running so late. I had a pretty sick boy at the end of the day, and I didn't want to leave until he was tucked in at the hospital. Hey – did you make this pumpkin pie?"

"No, sorry, I don't bake. Nettie brought that over along with some other food you'll get to sample over the next couple days."

"That's great! Nettie has such a kind heart. I wondered if she might do something like this. I'd forgotten how nice it is to have friendly neighbors. In the city you could drop dead in the street and people would just step right over you. How's Dad doing?"

"Fine. He's resting. Want me to warm up a plate for you?"

"Sure. I'll just go peek in on Dad and get rid of these books. Be right back."

Laura slipped her notes into the book and set it aside. By the time Bill returned, she had re-heated the stir-fry and set it on the table.

"Wow this is delicious," Bill said between mouthfuls. "I'm not used to home cooking. I've become well-acquainted with frozen meals and the microwave."

"It's nothing, really," Laura said. "Just a simple stir-fry."

"I appreciate it, nonetheless. Looks like Dad fell asleep in his chair. Anything new?"

"He's made decent progress. He still drags his right leg when he walks, but that's not surprising; however, with each day, he's getting more independent with his cane. I'm more concerned about his mood now than his physical recovery. When I don't have any specific activities for him, he just sits and stares out the window. He also doesn't seem to have an appetite and just picks at his food – it takes an hour for him to finish a meal."

Bill listened intently, keeping his gaze focused on Laura until she was finished. "What do you think it all means?" he asked.

"He's probably depressed. Perhaps we should have a psychiatrist evaluate him."

Bill cleared his plate and got up from the table. "That's a good suggestion," he said, while helping himself to some more stir-fry. "That would be a natural reaction. His patients are his life. He could overcome his weak arm and leg, but without speech, it would be hard for him to take care of anyone. Unless he finds another reason to live, he may not improve, but I'm not willing to give up on him yet."

"Good. Then we agree?" Laura asked.

Bill nodded in response. "There's a psychiatrist who helps us out periodically. I can get you her number."

"Wonderful. I'll call her in the morning," Laura said. She got up from the table and opened the refrigerator. "I'm in the mood for some Chardonnay. Care to join me?"

"Sure," said Bill, "but only one glass for me, in case I get paged."

"That's about all I can handle anyway," Laura said. "Like many Asians, I lack the alcohol dehydrogenase enzyme, so when I drink, my face turns beet red." She grabbed the bottle out of the fridge and wrestled the cork out. She poured Bill a glass and sat down with her own.

"How about a toast?" Bill said.

"Sure. To what?"

"A speedy recovery for Dad – and to what you've done to make it possible."

Laura's cheeks felt warm. She felt a little

embarrassed, but flattered, nonetheless. "To his recovery," she repeated quietly before taking a sip. The wine rolled smoothly off her tongue and warmed her chest as it went down.

"By the way," said Bill as he took a sip, "we haven't had much time to get to know each other. You haven't told me yet how you ended up here, in the middle of nowhere. Where are you from?"

"Are you sure you want to know? It's kind of boring."

"Not at all. I'm curious."

"Ok. I'm not sure I'd be willing to talk about this, but since you're plying me with alcohol, I'll try." She giggled, already feeling some effect of the wine. "I grew up in a one-room apartment in New York's Chinatown. My two younger sisters and I even shared a bed as kids until I was in junior high. We were poor, and I really wanted to get away. So, once I finished my nursing training, I took my first opportunity to flee. I've always dreamed of living in a tiny farmhouse in the Adirondacks. It's far enough from my parents, so they can't meddle in my activities, but close enough to visit them." Bill's intent eyes focused on her made her squirm a little. Was her face flushing due to his attention or from the wine? She took another sip.

"Saranac hospital seemed like a nice place to land," Laura continued. "There's enough going on in Saranac Lake, but it's still several hours from the city. But after two years emptying bedpans and answering the incessant rings of patient call buttons on the wards, I realized that an in-patient nursing career was not what I desired. So, that's why I'm here now. Sorry if I'm boring you."

"Not at all," said Bill. "It's funny, I grew up here, and couldn't wait to get to the city, and you did just the opposite. For some reason, we're never content with what we have. The 'grass is always greener elsewhere.'"

"True. So, I'm curious about the boy you admitted. What does he have?"

She listened intently, as Bill described Jeremy Whitman's illness.

"I've never seen a patient with chickenpox that severe before," Laura said.

"I've had a couple, but I'm not completely comfortable with my diagnosis, though. The distribution of the lesions wasn't typical, but they *did* look like early pox lesions. They also appeared to be in the same stage of development, which is odd. Usually with chickenpox, you get successive crops of lesions in different stages over time, but it may be too early to see that. I'm hopeful he doesn't have any undiagnosed immune compromising illness."

"Did you send any labs to confirm?" Laura asked.

"Yes - but those will take a couple of days or longer until I get the results. By then, his illness will probably have run its course. It may also be too early in the infection for any antibody tests to be positive." Bill held up his wineglass. "This isn't bad for 10 bucks a bottle."

They both laughed.

"Too bad medicine's not always straightforward," Laura said. "Guess that's why it's considered an art."

"Yeah," Bill said. "A fair amount of what I do is based on well-reasoned hunches, and consensus from a bunch of old guys sitting around a table. The next one or two days should tell me a lot more."

"True. Well, regardless of where you're practicing, I admire what you do. It's all fascinating," Laura said. "At one point, we thought we'd conquered infectious diseases, yet every month or two I read about some new emerging disease or an older disease resurfacing. I've been interested in medical history for some time. It's amazing how primitive some of our earlier attempts to treat disease were - like leeches and arsenic. We *still* have a long way to go."

"You can say that again," Bill said. "Did you ever think about going to medical school?"

"I guess if I could start over again I might consider it,

but I really like being a nurse. We really get to focus on our patients' daily needs. Besides, when I was growing up, my father believed in the traditional role of Chinese women: taking care of the home and the kids…and supporting the husband. In his generation, it was practically unheard of for a woman to have a career. I caused enough shock waves when I decided to go to nursing school."

"Why?"

"I'd rather not go into that," Laura said, realizing the wine was loosening her tongue. She drank only occasionally, so one glass made her light-headed. Bill didn't need to hear about her mother's harangues about why she wasn't married yet with three children. She recently had an argument with her mom about taking *this* job and leaving the city. How would she ever meet a nice young man in the boondocks?

A thumping sound came from the hallway as Alfred stumbled into the room with disheveled hair and wide eyes. His lopsided mouth opened as he struggled to speak, but no words came out.

"Dad, what is it?" Bill asked, as he jumped up from the table and grabbed his father's dangling right arm.

Alfred's face reddened and his neck veins swelled as if they would burst. More attempts to speak only produced a groan. Tears dripped down the side of his face.

"Take it easy, Dad."

Alfred pushed him away with his left hand and managed to blurt out "pa!" He lost his balance, spun around on his left leg in a pirouette that would have looked funny if he was 30 years younger. He landed with a loud whack as his left hand smacked the floor. Bill bent over to help him but was pushed away again.

"Laura, do you have any Haldol?" Bill called. "He'll stroke again if we don't calm him down."

"I'll get it." Laura immediately darted out of the room.

"Five milligrams!" Bill called after her. "Stat!"

Laura grabbed the medication from her kit and deftly

drew up the amount in a syringe before running back to the kitchen. Bill grabbed the syringe, rolled up Alfred's sleeve, and plunged the needle into his arm. Alfred made a few more attempts to rise, then gradually calmed down, and finally fell asleep.

"Let's get him back to his bed," Bill said. They carried him down the hallway to his bedroom.

"I've never seen him act like that," said Laura. "I'm glad you were here. What do you think got into him? Do you think he had a nightmare?"

"Beats me. I've had elderly patients before get very agitated and "sundown" at night."

They lifted him onto the bed and took his slippers off. Bill performed a quick physical assessment.

"I don't think he broke anything," he said, "and fortunately he didn't hit his head. We'd better let him rest now, but maybe when he wakes up he can communicate to us with a note what the problem was."

They turned and walked back down the hall to the kitchen.

"You think it was something we said?" Laura asked. "Was he listening to our conversation? What were we talking about?"

"I don't remember – your family?" Bill answered, "but I didn't know he was there until he practically fell into the room. Something scared him, though – I could see it in his eyes – but what?"

"I don't know," Laura said.

"I'll check on him in a few hours to make sure he's okay. You could probably use a break," Bill suggested.

"Thanks. I *am* pretty exhausted. Don't hesitate to wake me, though, if you need any help." Laura suddenly felt the weight of the long day on top of the effects of the wine. "I'll try to have him write something down for me in the morning."

10

May 19 (D+15)

Saturday morning's clinic schedule was particularly light, so Bill used the time to catch up, reviewing patient lab results, consultant referrals, x-rays, and annotating notes in patient charts. Rosemary had already left for the day, and Bill had already stopped by the hospital to check on Jeremy. His fever had come down a little, but his skin rash had blossomed, with more prominent lesions that had grown in size and quantity. Even after searching through a couple dermatology books and the latest in the medical literature, Bill didn't find anything that matched the appearance of the rash as closely as early chickenpox. It would take another day or two before he could be sure that the medicine was working.

Alfred was asleep when Bill left the house that morning around 7:00 a.m. Bill replayed in his mind the incident with Alfred the night before, but he still couldn't figure out what made him so agitated. Alfred's significant communication difficulties only compounded their previous tense relationship.

Bill had been so busy lately that he had not really had the chance to get acquainted with Laura, but last night was the first time he noticed how attractive she was, with her dark eyes, satiny ebony hair, and petite figure. In between patients he decided to give her a call.

"Hi, Laura. How's everything going there?"

"Good morning. We're managing. Alfred is awake. I gave him a pen and paper, but he hasn't shown any interest in communicating about what happened last night. I suspect he is upset about being sedated."

"I'm not surprised. He's probably having some challenges coping with all of this – it's happened abruptly, and he was completely functional and independent before the first stroke."

"Sure," said Laura, "it's not surprising. Something else about his demeanor has changed, though."

"Oh?"

"Yes. I think it's a positive development. He seems to have regained some *spark*, for lack of a better term. At one point, he indicated that he wanted me to get him some of his medical books. Now, instead of staring out the window, he's reading. I'm not sure what's gotten into him."

"Hmm, neither am I, but whatever the reason, that sounds like a good thing." Bill hesitated, a little nervous about his next question. "I was just thinking…I should be done with my charts soon. Any chance you could get someone to cover you for the afternoon?"

Bill held his breath in anticipation of her answer.

"Oh…uh…I don't know." She paused. "What's the matter?"

Bill feared he might have caught her off guard, but it was too late to quit.

"Oh, sorry. Nothing's the matter. It's just…since you're new to the area, I was wondering whether you might want to take a short hike. I know some great scenic lookouts nearby. What do you think?"

"Oh." The momentary silence on the line seemed endless. "It's pretty short notice." Another brief pause. Bill cursed himself for asking. "But since it's a weekend, my colleagues might have more flexible schedules. A couple of them owe me a favor. Tell you what. Let me make some phones calls. I'll call you back shortly."

"Great. Talk to you soon." Bill hung up the phone and clapped his hands together. At least it sounded like she was willing to consider the possibility.

Laura called back in fifteen minutes with good news: she'd found a substitute.

Norm Phinney hated to venture into the hospital on a weekend, but the fever had caused him to slip behind on his usual workload. He grabbed a cup of coffee from a vending machine and picked up his office mail. The usual familiar and welcome scent of formaldehyde in the morgue made him nauseated today, so he went to his office next door instead. His desk was covered with several stacks of unsorted papers, so he parked himself at an adjoining table and leafed through numerous pieces of junk mail and proceeded to open the various results sent from the small regional referral laboratory. He was particularly intrigued when he tore open the envelope holding the lab results from the samples he'd sent from the frozen body. The cultures that he'd incubated in his own lab had been contaminated with what appeared to be soil bacteria. The reference lab report noted similar results: *multiple bacterial and fungal organisms present, contamination suspected – recommend re-submission.* He wasn't surprised, especially given the body was covered in muck and ice when he received it, despite his attempt to obtain clean specimens. Every patient has different types of skin organisms, and soil is teaming with all types of bacteria and fungi. Getting a sterile sample off the skin of the frozen cadaver would be nearly impossible.

He turned to the next page of the lab report with viral culture results: *moderate growth. Forwarded to state reference lab in Albany for further testing. Final result pending.* Norm sat upright. The coffee churned in his stomach, and he felt a sense of foreboding. He hadn't expected viral growth. What could it mean? It wasn't unusual for the small regional laboratory he used to forward specimens to a more sophisticated reference lab with better equipment and testing capabilities, especially for virus identification. Doing additional tests was expensive and required specific expertise, which he didn't have.

Norm rubbed the rough scab on his left pinky. The

area was still sore, but improving, and the surrounding redness was gone, with the scab starting to contract. The bacterial laboratory culture was contaminated, so it wouldn't be surprising for Norm to infect himself with bacteria when he cut himself. The new antibiotic that Bill gave him probably helped, but he wondered whether it was possible that he inoculated himself with the same thing that was growing in the viral culture? What type of virus could make a similar kind of lesion? Herpes? CMV? Would a plant virus that survived in soil be able to infect an animal cell culture? He snatched the phone on his desk and punched in the numbers of the lab listed on the lab slip. After listening to 15 rings, he gave up, slamming the phone down and cursing the lab for not answering on the weekend.

He left his office hurriedly and strode into the morgue. The frozen body was still there. His attempts to identify it thus far were fruitless, but he had informed Sheriff Egglefield that there was nothing to indicate a suspicious death. The sheriff also had not found anything of concern for nefarious activity at the site where the body was recovered. Dental records could have helped, if the man lived originally in the local region. Unfortunately, it had been years since the town's dentist died, and any old records probably ended up in a dumpster. Without a relative to claim the body, soon he would have to sign it out as a John Doe.

Norm pulled on some gloves and walked to the wall of stainless-steel drawers. He yanked out the drawer with the cadaver. Staring down at the corpse again, the distribution of lesions now reminded him of some pictures of skin rashes he'd seen a long time ago. But where? Could he find those pictures again?

After examining the skin lesions again, Norm felt reassured that the small, brown lesions on the body that looked like deflated balloons bore no resemblance to the scab on his finger. He did another review through some of his medical texts, but he still couldn't find any pictures that looked even remotely like his scab.

Should he give Bill a call about the viral culture and bacterial contamination? What could he do about it, anyway? After all, Norm had nearly fully recovered from his infection, so what did it matter now? He decided not to make a big deal out of it and resolved to contact the reference lab on Monday.

As Bill climbed Owl's Head Mountain with Laura, he did his best to put thoughts of Jeremy Whitman out of his mind, but he always felt uneasy when he had a sick patient in the hospital. Laura kept at his heels the entire hike as they climbed over downed trees and skipped over tiny brooks en route to the summit. When they approached the higher elevations, the forest transitioned from oak, maple, and ash trees to evergreens, which progressively became shorter and scragglier. It was a beautiful day, and he enjoyed the crisp, clean air, and taking in the scent of pine. In addition to the usual birds chirping, he heard the occasional squirrel chatter and woodpecker hammering away at a tree trunk.

On the way up, Bill exchanged small talk with Laura about the weather, schools, and patient care. Laura stopped periodically to point out various medicinal plants she'd learned about from her grandfather. Bill grabbed her hand occasionally as they climbed over stumps, roots, and rocks.

Bill began to feel winded near the end of the climb as the air became thinner and felt ten degrees cooler than where they had parked at the base. Near the top they climbed the last several feet over rocks and boulders to reach the smooth granite peak, where they gazed at a magnificent, 180-degree panorama. The surrounding hills looked like a Monet painting with their spring colors coming into full bloom with speckles of green and occasional splashes of white and pink. Except for the occasional sound of an automobile engine floating up from the valley below, there was no way to tell they weren't the only two people on earth.

"Amazing," Laura said, as she gave a sweeping look around.

“Yeah,” Bill said. “Makes you feel like a king surveying your kingdom.”

Laura wore a thin white cotton sweater that contrasted nicely with her shiny black hair. She took off the knapsack she was carrying and whacked Bill lightly on the back with it.

"That's for making me the pack mule."

"Hey," Bill protested, “I did my share for the first half.”

“That was the *easy* part.”

“Ok,” Bill said, “if it’ll make you feel any better, I’ll carry it *all* the way down.”

“Great. Then it’ll be half empty.” Laura pulled out a water bottle and took a couple of sips. “So, any wild bears around here?” She handed a bottle to Bill, who took a gulp.

“Yeah. They’re around, and I’ve run into them occasionally, but they’re usually more afraid of us than we are of them. I’d be more worried about getting shot by a near-sighted hunter.”

The two of them sat on the edge of a rock ledge and split their homemade ham and cheese sandwiches and potato chips. Below them, the cliff dropped about 30 feet before meeting up with the forest.

"I haven't been up here in years," Bill said. "Dad used to take me here a lot when I was a kid. It's the perfect hike, because you get a rewarding view and it only takes a half-hour. This was a favorite hike of my college buddies when we used to take road trips up here.”

“Can you tell me about the different mountains we’re seeing?”

“I’ll try.” Bill gave her a tour of the horizon, pointing out the various peaks. Upper and Lower Wolfjaw and Sawteeth bore a resemblance to their names, with sharp, jagged, peaks. Giant, looked like the back of a large animal, and Gothics had a central rounded peak with two smaller side peaks and a concave center denuded by a rockslide – it bore the resemblance of a large church organ. Mount Marcy, the highest mountain in New York State, was a purple mound that peaked above some clouds far in the distance and had a much more gradual slope than the closer peaks.

"Teddy Roosevelt was hiking on Marcy when he learned that President McKinley had been shot," Bill said. "He had a harrowing trip through the mountains in the dark night, only to learn when he finally reached a train station that McKinley had already died."

Laura turned her attention to the valley that lay directly below them. "Looks pretty isolated down there."

"Yeah," Bill said. "Did you notice how treacherous some of those narrow roads were on our way out of the valley?"

Laura nodded.

"If we get a good blanket of snow or ice in the winter, it might be a couple days before anyone could plow through some of those mountain passes."

Nestled in the shadow of Upper Wolfjaw Mountain, Bill could barely make out a sliver of Glacier Lake. Even from this distance, he could distinguish the cooler end with a lighter color from a blanket of mist. Seeing the lake reminded him about the frozen corpse, so he told Laura all about the lake and the corpse, including Norm Phinney's sliced finger.

"Do you know what happened?" Laura asked.

"Norm's okay, but I don't know if he's figured out anything more from the autopsy." Bill then updated Laura on his pursuit of long-term care for his father. "Unfortunately, all the local facilities are booked solid. It could take months before something opens up."

"What are you going to do then?"

"I don't know. It is probably easier to find a place closer to me in Washington, DC, but I know he would object."

"Maybe you'll just have to stay here," Laura teased.

"It's crossed my mind. This place certainly has its rewards, but the medical care here is fairly routine. Plus, I'm just not excited about following in my dad's footsteps. We've had heated discussions over the years about how his medical practices are outdated, with his emphasis on physical diagnosis and he ignores the new technologies. I was trained to use the examination as a small part of the overall picture of the patient, and better incorporation of laboratory and other diagnostic tests."

"Which is better for the patients?" Laura asked.

"I like to think my approach is better. What do you think?" Bill asked.

"I guess you both bring complementary aspects to the bedside that can be beneficial. How close were you to him before the stroke?"

Bill frowned briefly, because her question was very perceptive.

"I'm sorry," Laura said. "I don't mean to pry." She patted Bill's arm lightly.

Bill fidgeted nervously before flinging a rock over the cliff. Several seconds later, they heard it crash against a rock somewhere below the forest canopy.

"That's okay," Bill said. "I don't mind." He sighed. "My mother died of breast cancer about 10 years ago. My dad had examined her and noticed a lump in her breast. He thought it was a benign cyst, so he didn't do any follow-up testing. When I heard about it 6 months later, I couldn't believe it. I insisted on a mammogram and biopsy, but by the time she had a complete workup, the cancer had already spread to her bones. To this day, I wonder whether an earlier mammogram would've helped, but it sure couldn't have hurt."

"I'm sorry," Laura said, as she looked down at the ground.

"Don't be." Bill said. "At this point, it is what it is. I hope I didn't upset you."

“No,” Laura said, as she turned her gaze toward the mountains on the horizon. Her eyes glittered in the setting sun. “But do you forgive him?” she asked, casting a sideways glance toward Bill.

“What do you mean?”

“Do you forgive him for his mistake?” Laura asked.

“Oh. I don’t know. I hadn’t really thought about it.”

“You might want to try,” Laura said as she patted his hand. “You might not have much more time.”

“Maybe,” Bill said as he wondered whether to reopen old wounds. He stood up and dusted off his pants. “We need to head back. The woods can turn dark very quickly as the sun sets. I’d also like to check on Jeremy Whitman before we go home.”

He grabbed Laura’s hand and helped her up. The sunset gave her cream-colored skin an orange glow.

As they repacked the knapsack and turned to leave, Bill noticed an awful odor. He turned to see a black bear blocking the center of the trail.

"Looks like we've got company,” Bill said, as he instinctively stepped between Laura and the bear. “Boy, you sure need a bath,” Bill said to the bear. He grabbed Laura’s hand, and tried to lead her around the bear, but the bear started moving toward them.

“Shouldn’t we play dead?” Laura mumbled while frozen in place.

“Too late for that,” Bill answered. "I think I know what he wants." Slowly, he pulled a loose branch from the ground, then he reached into the knapsack and handed Laura a leftover sandwich. “Here. When you throw the sandwich over there -” he gestured back toward where they had eaten - “I’m going to run at him with this stick. One, two, three, go!”

Laura threw the sandwich onto some rocks twenty feet away and Bill charged directly at the bear, screaming and waving his arms wildly. The bear was completely surprised and scrambled around him directly toward Laura.

In her haste to get away, Laura slipped on some pebbles and landed flat on her stomach. The bear continued to advance. Laura struggled to pull herself back up. Just as the bear was nearly upon her, Bill came from behind and whacked him square on the head. The bear stopped and snorted, before bounding off toward the sandwich. Bill rushed to help Laura to her feet.

"You okay?" he asked.

"Yeah. Thanks," she said breathlessly. "I'm shaken, and my heart's still pounding, but I'm okay. That was scary. I thought you said I didn't have to worry about bears?"

"That's what I thought," Bill said. "He's probably been fed by too many hikers and now expects a free meal. We're lucky he or she didn't have any cubs. That would've created a big problem. I'm just glad you're okay." Bill examined her hands and face closely for cuts. "I hope you don't get any bruises."

"I should be okay," she said. "If not, I'll go see a doctor. Know any good ones?"

"Very funny."

Laura laughed and patted Bill on the back. "Oh no," her tone changed. "Don't look now, but we have other company."

Sure enough, two bear cubs bounded up from the trail toward the larger bear.

"Shit!" Bill swore. "That probably *is* their mother." Fortunately, the large bear appeared content for now, munching on the sandwich in the distance, just as the two cubs sidled up to her.

"Let's get out of here before that mama bear turns on us again," Bill said.

He grabbed Laura's hand and the two of them darted down the rocky path, skipping over rocks and stumps on the way down. Bill occasionally let go of her hand and swung like Tarzan around the trunk of a small birch tree. When they reached the bottom, they were both breathing heavily.

"You feel like going somewhere for dinner?" Bill asked in between breaths. "After we drop by the hospital, there's a quiet place in the next valley, called the Elm Tree Inn."

"Sounds wonderful, as long as we're back before my substitute leaves around eight."

Just then Bill's beeper went off. He recognized the hospital number and pulled his cell phone out of the knapsack, but he couldn't get a good signal to call the hospital.

"The call's not going through," Bill said. "The cell service in these valleys is abysmal."

They got into the car and drove back toward Elizabethtown. On the way, Bill tried the number again. The phone rang ten times before an out-of-breath voice finally answered.

"In-patient ward."

"This is Dr. Denton. I was paged."

"Dr. Denton," the voice became frantic. "Thank God you called! It's Jeremy Whitman. He's coding!"

"Damn!" Bill felt as if someone kicked him in the stomach. "What happened?"

"I'll explain when you get here. Hurry!"

"I'm on my way." Bill jammed the accelerator to the floor making the tires screech as they headed into the mountain pass.

11

Jed Thorton could only pick at his burger and fries, so he set them aside, unable to finish his dinner. His muscles ached as he pushed away from the table. His red, bloodshot eyes burned as he looked around the blurred, sparse kitchen with its scuffed white linoleum floor and yellowed cream-colored walls. The room looked more barren than usual at night, as the meager light from a single fluorescent bulb lacked the strength to penetrate the darker recesses around him. His fiery throat, which had crept up this morning, worsened as the day progressed and helped to reduce his eagerness for food. His wife sat next to him and lit a cigarette, her face pale and blotchy without make-up and her dyed brown hair up in curlers. She wore a faded floral-patterned housecoat, which was threadbare in many places.

"Ain't you gonna finish, Hon?" she asked with an Adirondack drawl.

"No. I don't feel right," he answered.

"You're getting a pimple," she pronounced triumphantly, as if she'd made a great discovery. She leaned forward, smelling of stale smoke and beer as she analyzed the pimple. "My land, you've got a couple." She moved in for an even closer inspection, and the cigarette smoke floated into Jed's eyes.

"Get that smoke outta my face, woman! Damn!" Jed swore as he pushed her away.

"Why you so testy?" she asked defensively. "You need to see the doctor?"

"No. The smoke hurts my eyes. I told you, I just don't feel right, but no doctors," Jed said, rubbing his eyes.

Feeling transient muscle aches across his shoulders and back, Jed resisted the temptation to ask for a cigarette and instead pulled out a handful of chaw and stuffed it into his cheek, hoping it would soothe his burning throat. He got up from the table and burped before stepping onto the greasy tan shag carpet in the living room. He glanced in the mirror above the fireplace and noticed a couple small red spots on his cheeks. He dismissed them as nothing unusual, especially after a day in the sun. He turned the TV dial through the usual array of dull evening shows before he found a baseball game. Then he sunk into his easy chair, enjoying its comfortable embrace as he watched the game. The phone rang in the kitchen.

"Hey," his wife called. "Phone."

Jed reluctantly rolled out of his easy chair and stumbled back into the kitchen. He took the receiver from his wife.

"Yeah? Jed here."

"B…Boss?"

Jed recognized Scott Gurnsey's voice, although it sounded raspy and out of breath.

"Yeah, Scott, where've you been the last two days?" Jed asked. "Why haven't you called me?"

"Need help…come over?"

"What? What's going on?" Scott's mumbling began to ring alarm bells for Jed. "You sick?"

"Come over. Please?"

Jed looked at his watch. Eight o'clock - eight o'clock on a Saturday night. He had his heart set on baseball, but Scott was a good worker from out of town and he lived alone. Scott sounded like he was in trouble. Ever since his Army days, Jed prided himself on taking care of his men.

"You hang on son. I'm on my way." Jed put down the phone, suddenly forgetting about his aches and sore throat.

"What's up?" his wife asked.

"One of the boys sounds sick and needs help. I'm gonna check it out."

"I thought *you* was sick. You ain't goin' to one of those girly joints, are you?"

Jed ignored her, grabbed his hunting jacket, and left.

Scott lived in the hills outside the neighboring town of Keene Valley. Jed floored the accelerator down route 9N, reaching 80 miles per hour, until he had to slow down while descending two steep inclines between Elizabethtown and Keene Valley. On the ride over, Jed wondered what could be bad enough for Scott to miss work and then desperately call him. The whole damn construction schedule was falling apart, but he tried to ignore those concerns. Scott was a good boy, and Jed didn't want anything to happen to him.

As he swung up the dirt road to Scott's trailer, Jed barely missed a deer crossing the road. It stopped dead in its tracks, its eyes shining like two diamonds from the headlights. Jed slowed down, and the deer ran off, only to be followed by a second one that bounded right in front of his car. He drove slowly the rest of the way as the truck bounced and jerked over the road, scarred by water channels carved by the spring thaw.

When Jed arrived at the trailer, he knocked on the door, but there was no answer. Then he banged harder - still no answer. Jed walked around to the side of the trailer, and peered through the window, where sounds of the TV filtered out. He could see Scott lying on the couch. Jed banged on the window, but Scott didn't move. Back at the door, Jed jiggled the handle, but it was locked. He stood back, held his breath and kicked against the flimsy door, which popped open.

"Scott, it's me," Jed said, stepping inside.

Jed followed the sound of the television to the living room. The air in the house was stuffy and warm, and stunk like a locker room. Scott lay on the couch facing away from him, covered with a blanket. Jed shook him, but there was no response, so Jed turned him over. He gasped and drew back in horror as he saw Scott's face. He was barely recognizable, transformed by numerous boils filled with pus, like kernels of popcorn, which had exploded all over his face. He was mumbling to himself and breathing heavy and fast. Scott's skin burned hot to the touch and dripped with sweat, making his damp clothes stick to his body.

"You need a doctor," Jed said, grunting as he picked up the thin boy and hoisted him over his shoulder in a fireman's carry. Once at the car, he laid the boy down in the back seat, and panted in the front seat from exhaustion, breathing through his mouth, which made his sore throat burn like it was being stuck with a red-hot poker. When he finally caught his breath, he threw the truck into gear and jammed his foot on the accelerator, heading down the hill toward the closest clinic in Keene Valley.

12

Bill rushed in through the back entrance of the 10-bed inpatient ward past white cinder block walls tinged an eerie yellow by incandescent ceiling bulbs. Multiple hospital staff stood gawking outside a room at the end of the hall, like bystanders witnessing a car wreck - the cardinal sign of a patient in trouble. Bill stopped a moment to catch his breath before elbowing his way through the crowd into the steamy room. He immediately recognized two poor prognostic signs: the stench of burnt flesh, caused by the electrical defibrillator, and the raw meaty odor of fresh blood.

"Anyone who doesn't need to be here should leave immediately," Bill said loudly as he gestured for people to clear out. The vultures hovering near the door reluctantly began to slide away.

Jeremy's naked, bloated form lay on the bed in the center of the room, his red-streaked sunken, vacant eyes staring at the ceiling. A surreal rainbow of colored wires, each with its own purpose, snaked from pads on his chest to a heart monitor near the head of the bed. A nurse leaned over the boy, rhythmically pumping on his chest causing the bedsprings to squeak with each futile thrust. A respiratory therapist stood at the head of the bed forcing oxygen into Jeremy's lungs with every squeeze on a plastic Ambu-bag in syncopation with the chest compressions. Clear fluid hanging in plastic IV bags above the bed dripped continuously into intravenous lines that weaved and intertwined with one another down into the boy's arms and legs.

Jeremy's deathly gray skin was punctuated by the numerous pus-filled bumps Bill had seen before, but now, large purple and red bruises had blossomed around those bumps, like spilled paint spreading on the floor. Streams of blood flowed crimson out of Jeremy's nostrils, charting the curves of his face and down his neck. Pink, foamy fluid gurgled up into the endotracheal tube in between each squeeze on the Ambu-bag. The staff stepped around dark red sticky blood pools that had congealed on the floor. Stained glove prints were amplified on starched white sheets like blood on newly fallen snow.

Bill recognized Mrs. Whitman, cowering in the corner of the room, her face a ghostly pale and her eyes transfixed in horror.

"Move her out of here, NOW!" Bill yelled at the closest nurse, while gesturing toward the frightened mother. The nurse jumped in surprise, but then immediately understood the situation and led the distraught mother outside.

Standing to the left of the bed, Bill recognized Joel Brown, the contract doctor who frequently worked in the emergency room. He periodically barked a medication order to one of the nurses in between reviewing the heart rhythm strip. His pale green scrubs looked like someone had finger-painted on them with blood. Tight lines in the corners of his mouth relaxed when he noticed Bill.

"Hey, Bill" Joel said. "Glad you're here."

"What happened?" Bill asked.

"The nurse on duty found him seizing and called a CODE. By the time I got here, he was as cyanotic as a Smurf. I tube'd him immediately, but he already had some large oral bruises and probably aspirated blood. When we got his clothes off, we noticed all these other ecchymoses, in addition to his baseline rash," he gestured toward some larger reddish/purplish areas with bleeding under the skin. "He's oozing everywhere."

"So I see," Bill said. "The ecchymoses are new since this morning. His platelet count was slightly low, but not bad enough to cause this."

"Continue CPR." Brown gestured to the nurse on the bed.

"My arms are about to give out," the nurse complained.

"Jackie," Brown said, gesturing to a nursing assistant standing by. “Take over compressions." The assistant switched places with the nurse and began the rhythmic up and down motions on Jeremy’s chest.

"What have you done since you intubated him?" Bill asked.

"By the time we hooked up the monitor, his heart rhythm was already flat line,” Brown said. “We've gone through the whole algorithm: oxygen, epinephrine, amiodarone, atropine. Now I'm trying escalating epinephrine doses. We shocked him a couple times in case he was in fine v. fib, but it didn’t do any good. I sent some blood gases. His oxygen’s in the doghouse and his acidosis is getting worse. I transfused him a couple units of packed red blood cells and FFP to try and shore up the blood loss. I’m not sure what else to do."

Ventricular fibrillation, “v. fib,” was incompatible with life and meant the heart was quivering, like a bag of worms. The acidosis meant the cells in Jeremy’s body were starving for oxygen.

"Sounds like you've done the right things," Bill said as he moved closer to the bed.

At this point, Jeremy’s chance of surviving was infinitesimal. Bill needed to make sure that nothing had been overlooked, because something minor could mean the difference between life and death.

"Hold chest compressions," Bill said.

The nursing assistant stopped her rhythmic pushing. Bill felt at Jeremy’s neck for the carotid artery but couldn’t detect any pulse. With his stethoscope, he strained his ears to listen for a heartbeat, but all he could hear was the crackling of Jeremy’s lungs with each squeeze of the Ambu-bag.

"The tube’s in the right place," Bill said. "Resume chest compressions.” He hung his stethoscope back around his neck.

Bill fiddled with each of the wires attached to the

heart monitor to ensure none were disconnected. Fresh blood coated the inside of Jeremy's right eye, making it glow like something out of a horror film. His wide, empty pupils, like dark tunnels, didn't constrict as Bill shined a pen light into them one at a time. The absence of a pupillary reflex could've been caused by atropine, but more likely indicated Jeremy was brain dead. Even so, Bill didn't want to give up quite yet. He flipped the knobs on the heart monitor several times to evaluate different EKG leads, but there was no evidence of heart activity.

"Since he's been bruising, it would be good to ensure he doesn't have cardiac tamponade due to bleeding in the pericardium." Bill put on some sterile gloves and turned to one of the nurses. "Hand me a long 18-gauge needle and a 50-milliliter syringe."

The nurse opened them one at a time so that Bill could grab them and maintain sterility. Once he twisted the needle onto the syringe, he wiped an area on the left side of Jeremy's central chest with Betadine. Then he slowly inserted the needle below and to the left of the breastbone, while pulling back on the syringe plunger. He felt a pop as the needle entered the pericardial sack, which surrounds the heart. He pulled even harder on the syringe plunger, hoping that blood or fluid would fill the syringe, because fluid in the sack would prevent the heart from pumping blood. No fluid came back, though, so he removed the needle and syringe and discarded them.

Bill stood back, took a deep breath, and choked back a sob. "Resume compressions," he said. He let the CODE continue for a few more minutes with a couple more rounds of medicines, hoping for some miracle. Despite all the medications and perspiration being expended in the room, Jeremy remained deathly gray.

"How long has this been going on?" Bill asked.

"We started a 5:15," said a nurse holding a clipboard. "The time is now -" she glanced down at her watch - "6:30."

"He's gone," Bill whispered partly to himself and partly to Dr. Brown. "Does anyone have any objection to calling the CODE?" Bill asked loudly. The others in the room sullenly shook their heads. Bill gestured to Dr. Brown to end the code.

"Call the CODE," Brown said.

"Time of death: 6:30," the nurse with the clipboard said.

Bill removed and discarded his gloves before washing his hands. "Thanks for the help," Bill said, as he patted Brown on the arm. He turned to the nurse with the clipboard. "Please move Mrs. Whitman into the quiet room. I'll be there in a minute."

"Yes, Doctor. Give us about 20 minutes to clean up the room, and then we can let her back in." She gestured to the other room attendants to start cleaning up.

"Okay. Thanks."

Bill left the humid, suffocating room and welcomed stepping into the cooler hallway air. He washed his hands and face vigorously in the bathroom, as if he could somehow rinse away the death. The water dripped off his face as he leaned over the sink while reliving the CODE in his mind and thinking about the first time he saw Jeremy the day before. Could he have done something different to change the outcome? How many times had he done this before? It was one thing to inform the family when an elderly person died, but when it was a child, there were no words that could be consoling.

Bill grabbed a paper towel and dried his face and hands. In the dimly lit bathroom mirror, bloodshot eyes stared back at him, and he noticed for the first time some creases at the corner of his eyes. Years of nights like this were taking their toll.

He left the bathroom and walked slowly and deliberately down the hall. A deathly hush had settled over the hospital staff – they, too, were feeling the trauma.

The quiet room at the corner of the emergency room was tiny with green wallpaper to give a feeling of intimacy and calm for those grieving. But like the rest of the hospital, the room hadn't been modernized since the 1970s and now the furniture looked cheap and inadequate.

Mrs. Whitman sat on a worn green sofa, with puffy, red eyes and a face streaked with tears. A nurse consoled her, with an arm around her shoulders. Mrs. Whitman looked up, with hopeful eyes, when Bill entered the room. He sat in a chair across from her.

"Mrs. Whitman," he whispered. "I'm sorry…Jeremy's gone." He stopped to let his words sink in.

"No!" She buried her head in the nurse's shoulder.

Despite all she had seen that evening, Bill knew she still hoped his words would be different. He also knew that the trauma would erase most of what he said from that point on.

"Would you like me to call your husband?"

"He's not home," she said in between sobs. She took out a tissue from her purse and dabbed her eyes and nose. "He's still on a school field trip with our daughter in Washington, DC. I'll call him as soon as I can."

"Can I call the chaplain for you?"

"Yes. Thank you."

"Is there anything else I can do for you?"

"Why, doctor? Tell me…why? Jeremy was healthy. He played sports. He was a good student. How could he get chickenpox? He had the vaccine."

"I know. I don't understand it either. Some things I just can't explain. I'm so sorry." Bill waited for a moment, then broached the subject he always dreaded, but he knew was necessary. "Mrs. Whitman, I know this is a very difficult time to ask you, but I need your permission to have an autopsy performed."

"What?" She looked incredulous. "Not on your life!"

"We use the autopsy to better understand how this

happened. It might be the only way we can."

"No. I won't let you. Leave me alone…please."

"I understand. I'm sorry, Mrs. Whitman. Please let me know if you change your mind. Again, I'm so sorry." Mrs. Whitman didn't respond but put her face in her hands and continued sobbing.

Bill got up slowly and opened the door. He signaled to the nurse that he would call the chaplain, before he closed the door quietly.

Bill stood outside the door momentarily, relieved to be out, but frustrated about the autopsy. There was never really a good time to ask about it, especially after an unexpected death. Some deaths, like Jeremy's, naturally saddened and perplexed him. Did Jeremy die because he hadn't made the right diagnosis, or hadn't gotten the right treatment to him in time? If he could figure that out, perhaps if a similar patient ever came along, even years from now, he might manage the patient differently. The autopsy was the final chance for the dead to teach the living.

Down the hall at the nurses' station, Bill called the Chaplain, then he sat down and grabbed a piece of paper and pen. He reviewed the CODE paperwork. Only rarely had he seen someone bleeding so profusely, usually only in patients with liver failure from alcohol-induced cirrhosis or hepatitis, with their livers so eaten away that they no longer produced important clotting factors. But this was a healthy child. The disease ravaged Jeremy so abruptly, Bill had to consider other possibilities. Perhaps he didn't have chickenpox at all. Mrs. Whitman's question echoed again in his mind. *How could he get chickenpox? He had the vaccine.*

Bill pulled Jeremy's chart from the wall rack, and he wrote a note describing the CODE, then he filled out a draft death certificate. He returned to Jeremy's room with several needles and syringes. The room now smelled of disinfectant, and the nurses were just about done with the cleanup. A lonely white sheet on the bed silhouetted Jeremy's motionless corpse. In a short time, the blood would be clotted and more difficult to obtain for further laboratory studies, so Bill put on some gloves, lifted the sheet, and swabbed the child's groin area with an alcohol pad. He inserted the needle into Jeremy's groin and watched dark red, purple-tinted blood fill the syringe as he pulled back on the plunger. He removed the needle and placed a gauze pad over the groin. Then he stuck the needle into assorted blood sample bottles and tubes. The blood hissed as the vacuum containers pulled the blood through the needle and into each container. Back at the nurses' station Bill handed the containers to a nurse.

"Send the red-top tubes for titers of varicella (chickenpox), herpes simplex, and Rocky Mountain spotted fever. Send the bottles for aerobic and anaerobic blood cultures, including meningococcus."

The nurse got out a pen and wrote the orders down.

"Thanks," said Bill. "Anything I can help you with?"

"I think we've got everything under control," she answered. "The chaplain should be here in about fifteen minutes. I'll take care of the remaining paperwork. You can sign the official death certificate when the admin guys come in on Monday."

The tubes and bottles clinked into one another as Bill put them into plastic bags. Then he removed his gloves and washed his hands in the sink behind the nurses' station. Only then did he realize how exhausted he was. It was already 8 p.m.

As he headed back down the corridor toward where he entered, he noticed Laura sitting on a bench at the end of the hall. He closed his eyes and chastised himself for forgetting about her.

"Laura, I am *so* sorry. I got caught up in the CODE and completely forgot..."

"That's okay," she interrupted. "You were obviously tied up. I always carry something to read. I called my sub, so she knows I'll be late. What happened?" She put her book into her purse and stood up.

"I prefer not to talk about it right now," Bill said as he held her arm. “It’s probably too late now to go out for dinner, so let’s go home and I’ll be content with leftovers. I don’t have much of an appetite anymore anyway."

13

Bill and Laura drove home in silence. The porch light cast a haunting yellow glow in an arc over the front of the house as they drove up the driveway. Large moths swarmed around the light in a frenzy, like bees around a hive. The sound of Roaring Brook, usually prominent on a quiet night, seemed unusually muffled this evening. Once they were inside, Bill checked on his dad, who was already asleep, while Laura released her substitute. They converged in the kitchen and put together a quick dinner from the collection of food from the neighbors.

At first, Bill didn't want to discuss the CODE, but Laura's profound interest helped him overcome his reluctance. He gave her a play-by-play account of what happened to Jeremy, from the moment he first met him until the CODE was called.

"What about the possibility that this wasn't chickenpox?" Laura asked. "That would explain why the vaccine didn't protect him." Laura finished her meal and pushed her plate away.

"I know," Bill said as he scratched his head, "I've been wrestling with that. Before I left the hospital, I drew some blood for cultures and antibody tests. Hopefully those results will give me better insight into what happened, but the problem is, the kinds of diseases that make someone bleed like Jeremy generally don't occur around here, except for maybe meningococcus or Rocky Mountain spotted fever. Jeremy hadn't traveled anywhere. If he picked up some exotic disease like Ebola from Africa, then someone else must have infected him. But who? How?"

Bill got up from the table and put his dishes in the sink and washed them. He dried his hands and turned back to Laura.

"Is that enough dinner for you? We can scrape up

something else if you want."

"No thanks," Laura said, smiling. "I'm fine."

"Anyway," Bill sat back down at the table, "I'll do some more research tonight and see what else I can come up with. By the way, did your substitute have any problems? Dad seemed okay when I checked on him."

"Nothing concerning. In fact, he seemed pretty content even before we went hiking."

At that moment, a tapping noise sounded from the hallway and a moment later, Alfred hobbled into the kitchen wearing in his pajamas. He opened his crooked mouth and attempted to speak but only grunted. As he strained to speak, his face reddened, and his neck veins bulged. He held up his left hand and pointed at his right upper arm, but he nearly fell before steadying himself with his cane. Bill got up from the table, fearing another episode like last night, but Alfred gave up, shook his head, turned and hobbled away. Bill followed him down the hall.

"Dad? What is it? Does your arm hurt?"

Alfred sat down on his bed and shook his head. Bill put his hand on Alfred's right arm. He slid up Alfred's sleeve and looked for any sign of injury. Not seeing anything, he pulled the sleeve back down. Alfred waved Bill away with his left hand. Bill grabbed a piece of paper and pen off the desk in Alfred's study and put them on his father's lap.

"Dad. Tell me what's going on. Write something down."

Alfred just sat there shaking his head. Bill gave up and returned to the kitchen.

"Any luck?" Laura asked.

"No, but I'm worried about him," Bill said. "It seems like he really wants to tell us something important. But what? Why was he pointing at his arm?"

"He was certainly animated," Laura said, excitedly. "You don't think he's starting to consider he might work again, do you?"

Bill thought for a moment before responding.

"I don't know. He *has* made significant progress. I must admit that I was a little surprised to see him walking with just that cane. It would be wonderful if he recovered, but let's be realistic. The odds are low unless he can communicate. He's had a pretty big stroke."

"But what *is* it about us being in the kitchen?" Laura said, throwing up her arms. "Was he eavesdropping on us again? What were we talking about this time?"

"I don't know." Bill rubbed his chin and thought for a moment. "We were talking about Jeremy. Hmm. Last night we were –"

"- The same thing." Laura said and slapped her hand on the table. "We were talking about Jeremy."

"Really?" Bill knitted his eyebrows. "Are you sure?"

"Yes. Remember? You told me you were testing Jeremy for herpes and chickenpox."

"Damn!" Bill said. "You don't think he has a hunch about what it is, do you?"

Laura shrugged. "Maybe."

"I'm going to ask him," Bill said. He got up and walked briskly down the hall to Alfred's room. Alfred was asleep. Disappointed, Bill returned to the kitchen.

"He's asleep," Bill said. "I don't want to wake him and get him agitated again. Do me a favor, though. I'll be gone in the morning by the time he wakes up. See if you can coax something out of him."

"I'll try."

The kitchen light reflected in Laura's eyes. Despite all the evening's tragic events, Bill couldn't help but notice Laura's beautiful, full red lips squeezed together into a slight pout.

Bill's beeper sounded and pulled him out of his musing. He frowned when he read the number on the beeper.

"It's the Emergency Room," Bill said. "Haven't we had enough excitement for one evening?" He got up and grabbed the phone.

"Maybe it's about the death certificate?" Laura asked as she got up from the table and put her dishes in the sink.

"Doubtful," said Bill as he punched in the ER numbers. "They wouldn't page me at this hour for that. Besides, the nurse already told me she'd have the official one ready for signature on Monday."

Dr. Brown at the hospital answered the phone.

"Hi Joel, Bill Denton here. I was paged."

"Thanks for responding, Bill." Brown then described a five-year-old girl with a temperature of 104 degrees.

"Any source for the fever?" Bill asked.

"Nothing yet. No pneumonia. No diarrhea. Her throat and ears look clean."

"How about her urine?"

"Nothing on the urinalysis, but her BUN and creatinine are elevated."

Bill felt a knot in the pit of his stomach, as a ready source of the girl's infection appeared elusive. An elevated BUN and creatinine could indicate she was dehydrated but could also be a harbinger of something worse: kidney failure.

"Oh, yeah," Brown said. "She has a rash--"

"What!" Bill said, feeling a surge of adrenaline. "There's your fever source. Why didn't you tell me that up front?"

Laura looked up from the dishes and raised her eyebrows.

"Sorry, pal," Brown said, "I'm juggling a couple other patients, and it slipped my mind. Looks like it could develop into chickenpox – tiny fluid-filled vesicles mostly on her face right now. I thought about sending her home with a diagnosis of chickenpox, but the high fever worried me, especially after tonight's CODE. D'you mind coming back in to check her out, in case she needs to be admitted?"

"Is she stable?"

"Yes. Her pulse is elevated, about 110, probably from

the fever, but blood pressure and respirations are okay."

"Good. I'll be there shortly. Oh -- one more thing. Has she ever received the chickenpox vaccine?"

"Yeah, I saw it in her shot record."

"Hmm," said Bill. "It'll take me about fifteen minutes to get there. Depending on how sick she looks, we may want to transfer her to Saranac Lake rather than admit her here."

Bill hung up the phone. He felt a little light-headed.

"Bill," Laura said, "you look like you've just seen a ghost."

"Maybe I have."

"Why don't you sit down?"

"Good idea." Bill sat down at the table and began to feel better.

"Here," said Laura, "have some water."

As he drank the water, Bill described the girl's status. "And get a load of this – she's had the chickenpox vaccine."

Laura dropped a pan, which clattered in the sink, startling both of them.

"Sorry. But that sounds like Jeremy," Laura said, her eyes widening.

"I know," Bill said. "That's what concerns me. Two vaccinated kids a day apart, with what looks like chickenpox. I shouldn't jump to conclusions, though. I'll have to examine her and make an assessment." Bill got up from the table. "Listen, I'll probably be gone for several hours. I -" he hesitated for a moment –"I really enjoyed spending the afternoon with you. I'm sorry I have to go. I would've liked to talk more."

"It's okay," Laura said, smiling, "I'll be around. Would you like some coffee for the road?"

"No thanks. I'm already pumped full of adrenaline." Before leaving, Bill grabbed a soda out of the refrigerator. "See ya," he said and waved.

"Hey, Bill," Laura called after him, grinning, "small town medicine's not so dull lately, is it?"

14

May 20 (D+16)

Somewhere lost in a dream, Bill watched his father tapping his knuckles on the kitchen table, telling Bill the elusive diagnosis was at his fingertips. “Wake up,” Alfred said.

Bill opened his eyes and his bedroom came slowly into focus around him. Again, he heard the knuckle-tapping sound from his dream, but he realized instead that someone was knocking on his bedroom door.

“Yes?” he mumbled hoarsely.

"Hey, sleepyhead,” Laura’s muffled voice sounded from the hallway. “Rise and shine."

Bill rolled over. "Tell me it's not the morning already," he pleaded.

"It's already ten o'clock," Laura said. "I made you some breakfast. Come on down when you’re ready."

Bill remembered the mounds of work he had to do and gave up on any more sleep.

“Ok, thanks,” he said. “I’ll be down in a minute.”

Bill heard Laura’s footsteps fading down the hallway. He got out of bed and stumbled into the shower. The steamy water helped to revitalize both his mind and body. He stared at the water swirling down the drain, feeling the water cascade over his back, and he couldn’t help but think about his ex-wife. After a fight, they often ended up in the shower together. She always complained that he wouldn’t share his true feelings, but Bill had spent years before they met perfecting the ability to remain emotionally detached and calm in a crisis. What worked in the hospital didn’t work at home. His wife’s desire for more intimacy and his resistance had destroyed the marriage.

Over the years, he’d become accustomed to living

alone, but Laura's presence reminded him how nice it was to have a female around for conversation and friendship, especially someone who understood medicine. His ex-wife had been a schoolteacher, so it was hard for her to understand the challenges he faced every day in the hospital.

After showering and shaving, Bill dressed with urgency, but still ensured he squared away every button and that his tie could pass a military inspection. Old habits die hard. The wooden floor creaked as he stepped into the hallway and ran down the stairs toward the kitchen. On the way, he passed his father's room and was surprised to see that his bed was empty – a good sign.

Laura sat at the table in the kitchen reading the Sunday paper.

"That was quick," she said. "I thought for sure I'd have to go back in there and light some firecrackers. What time did you get in?"

"Around 4:00 am, but thanks for waking me. I wasn't sleeping well anyway. I've got to figure out what's going on with these children. It's going to take some phone calls and extensive literature review."

Bill didn't sit down, but ate quickly while standing, wolfing down the bacon and eggs Laura made. He slowed down some with a cinnamon roll but drained his coffee with a few gulps. He grabbed the kitchen door handle and prepared to leave.

"That was fast," Laura said. "Before you go, can I make you some more coffee for the road?"

"No thanks. I apologize for rushing, but I really need to get moving."

Laura frowned. "But can you at least tell me what happened with the girl last night?"

Bill gave in to her curiosity but didn't sit down.

"Ok, but I'll be quick. She was severely ill, like Jeremy, with a rapid pulse and respiratory rate, and a rash on her face and extremities. Her rash was even more prominent than Jeremy's. Given what happened to Jeremy, I felt the urgency to move her to a better hospital with intensive care assets, so I accompanied her in the ambulance to the ICU in Saranac Lake. I'm worried, because she appeared to be spiraling downhill when I left, but I'm hoping that she has a better chance in that monitored setting than here in E'town. Fingers crossed."

"That's really scary," Laura said. "How will you find out what happened to her?"

"I had an extensive discussion with the pediatric intensivist on call. He promised to update me regularly on her progress. Apparently, they haven't seen anything like this lately."

Bill grabbed the door handle to leave.

"I'm not surprised," Laura said. "Feel free to call later and I'll let you know how Alfred's doing."

"Great," Bill said, looking forward to that conversation. He opened the door. "By the way, thanks for breakfast."

"Sure." Laura smiled.

Bill raced into town. It was a luxury being able to speed down the country roads without traffic or a speed limit. In Washington, DC, even on a Sunday morning, he would be honking his way through the usual beltway gridlock.

As he entered his father's medical clinic, he rushed by walls in the office that charted his father's education, displaying diplomas from Elizabethtown High School, college, medical school, internship, and residency. On one wall hung a map of Africa – a remnant from his dad's years in the Peace Corps, and behind the desk sat a bookshelf next to a large window. In one corner sat a box, where Bill piled together all his father's medical instruments. With his father's return to work now unlikely, he wasn't sure what to do with them.

Bill raised the window blinds and opened the window, pausing for a moment to let the air and sunlight stream in. The morning breeze felt refreshing on his face, although it carried with it the scent of cow manure. He envied the cows, as they rested on the grass in the distant pasture chewing their cud, oblivious of any concerns.

Bill worried about the possibility that there could be more sick kids out there. He turned away from the window, called and left a phone message at the school for the principal to be on notice for kids with rashes. There were probably two-to-three weeks left in the school year. For an outbreak of something like chickenpox, summer vacation might be the right prescription to reduce close contact between the kids and decrease the spread of disease.

Next, he left a message at Mayor O'Donnell's office briefly describing his concerns that an outbreak might have begun. If the mayor had seen Rosemary recently, she might already have told him about Jeremy's hospitalization, but she wouldn't have heard yet about Felicia Jamison, the five-year-old girl from last night, or possibly even Jeremy's death.

The large medical textbook that Bill pulled off the shelf landed with a thud as he dropped it on the desk. The publication date was current enough to satisfy him. He leafed through the index for *vesicles (skin)* and turned to the appropriate pages. He found a table that listed several diseases. Pulling out a pen and a pad of paper from the desk to take notes, he wrote *Differential Diagnosis: Vesicular Rash* at the top of the page, followed by the diseases listed: *chickenpox, herpes simplex, smallpox, vesicular rickettsiosis.* He also listed *drug reactions* and *insect bites*, since they might mimic other conditions. After reading through the book for a moment, he made some notes next to each of the listings:

1) Chickenpox (varicella) - may be deadly in neonates and adults.

2) Herpes simplex - generally localized, may be deadly in immunocompromised.

3) S*mallpox – eradicated, 1980.*

4) *Vesicular rickettsiosis - generally mild,*

transmitted by mites; no reported deaths.

5) *Drug reactions - what about vaccines?*

6) *Insect bites - could the children have had insect exposure?*

He was reassured to read that chickenpox could cause hemorrhaging in severe cases. That made it still the most likely diagnosis. After reading some more, he pushed the textbook aside, then folded up the piece of paper and shoved it into his pocket. He then did a search on Pub Med and the Internet to see if there were any recent outbreak reports. Nothing, but the Internet modem dial up was slow and he couldn't get some of the website information to load. The county health department might be interested in hearing about these cases. He dialed a number listed in the phone book, but there was no answer. On the bookshelf, he found the yellow international travel and immunization guidebook from the Centers for Disease Control and Prevention (CDC), which listed a telephone number for consultations, so he tried it. After an endless series of recorded menus that took him in circles, he finally gave up.

Frustrated that no one else seemed to work on Sunday, he didn't think his investigative work could wait until Monday. He had never done an outbreak investigation, since that was usually the purview of the epidemiologists and public health departments. Where should he begin? It would be nice to talk to someone with a little more experience who could give him some insight.

He picked up the phone and dialed a number in Maryland. He hadn't spoken with his old Army buddy, Dr. Luis Martinez, in a while, but he thought he still remembered his number. Maybe he could help. They had met as family practice residents and afterward Martinez had channeled his career into public health.

The last he'd heard, Martinez was still working at the Army bioweapons defense lab, USAMRIID, the U.S. Army Medical Research Institute of Infectious Diseases at Fort

Detrick, just outside Washington, D.C. Martinez was a workaholic, so he wouldn't be surprised to find him in the office or the lab on a Sunday. As he listened to the phone ring, he envisioned Martinez with his thick head of black hair and black bushy moustache.

"Colonel Martinez here. This line is unsecure."

Bill recognized the cheery voice with the slight Hispanic accent.

"Hey doc." Bill falsely lowered his voice and added a gruff tone, imitating one of their former patients.

"Damn. Bill Denton, is that you? You *dog*! What are you up to?"

"Martinnnnez," Bill teased. "More than I care to admit." Bill updated him on his temporary move to the Adirondacks. "I'm glad to see my tax dollars are being spent well - seems like no one else works on the weekends. How is Uncle Sam treating you?"

"You know the old saying," Martinez responded, "pass the buck, shoot the shit, and get a receipt. But seriously, I finally got some traction for my international surveillance system that leverages the overseas military lab network. I've got more work than I can handle, which is a good thing. I can't remember the last time we talked. You haven't sent me a Christmas card in at least a decade."

"Come on – it's only been 3 years," Bill said. "I know, because Susan used to do the cards, and we've been divorced for about that long."

"Gee, Bill, I'm sorry to hear about Susan, although I remember things were rocky between you two when we were in Somalia together. Linda's been threatening to leave me for years, but now that I'm a Colonel, the Army's finally stopped moving us every two years, and she seems a little happier."

"Maybe it's because your pension will be worth more now that you're a 'bird' Colonel. Better to hang in there rather than divorce you."

"Maybe," Martinez said, letting out a hearty laugh.

“The pay is definitely a little better than when I was a lowly major, but it also comes with a lot more headaches. Anyway, to what do I owe this honor?”

Bill explained the situation with the two children. "I was hoping you could guide me through what is starting to look like a public health disaster, and how to conduct an outbreak investigation."

"I see why you're concerned,” Martinez said. “It's funny that you called today. I write this global disease report four times a year, and I was just looking at the latest varicella numbers. We don’t really track varicella, because it’s not a reportable disease in the military or with the CDC, but the little data that I have shows a rise in the number of varicella cases in the U.S. this quarter. That seems unusual now that we have a vaccine; I would expect to see a decline instead.”

“Is it possible that more docs are reporting it, simply *because* it’s becoming less common?” Bill asked.

“That’s certainly possible,” Martinez responded. “Regardless, those unusually severe cases you’re seeing could be the canary in a coal mine, as a harbinger of a bigger problem on the way. Two really sick kids in such a small town points to an epidemic until proven otherwise. If you can catch it early and intervene, maybe you can mitigate a potential disaster.”

"I’m glad you share my concern. So, let’s say this *is* the beginning of an epidemic, what next?"

"For any outbreak investigation," Martinez said, “we follow the same general approach. Start with a case definition - the symptoms and physical signs that define the illness. In this situation, something like fever and rash might work. Then look for other patients who fit your case definition. Since only the sickest patients seek medical care, chances are there could be other ill people in the community, but you just haven’t heard about them - yet. Contact the parents of those two sick children and ask them about the things the kids have been doing or may have had in common. Look for something –

anything - which links them to each other. Having received the chickenpox vaccine already doesn't help, unless there were a bad batch of vaccine, because most kids that same age would have received the vaccine. Most likely it means that this probably isn't chickenpox. You really should canvass the community to find other cases. Also, keep the local government in the loop. They can help you share important information with the community."

"I've already left messages with the school principal and the mayor," Bill said.

"You see, buddy, you're ahead of the game. You don't need my help at all."

"I wish I felt that way," Bill said.

"Have you hooked up with the county health department?"

"Not yet. I called them, but there's no answer. I've heard they're short-staffed from budget cuts. How about the CDC?"

"Too early to involve them. They'll just turf you back to the local or state guys. The CDC won't help you unless this spreads to multiple states or the locals call them in."

Bill jotted down highlights of Martinez's recommendations. He felt a breeze come through the window, which ruffled the multiple papers sitting on his desk.

"So, what else?" asked Bill, poised to scribble some more notes.

"Find those additional cases and it can help you figure out how this thing spreads. Once you have that, stopping it is easy. Well, maybe not easy, but possible."

"Yeah. That doesn't sound easy."

"Really - it's that simple," Martinez said. "Can you believe they pay me to do that? And while you're at it, once you know what's going on, engage with the media. You'll want to shut down rumors before they start. Be as candid with them as you can. In fact, if you flood them with information, they'll probably leave you alone."

“I get the point,” Bill said.

"Good. Oh, and one final thought: sometimes the most important clue to the cause of an outbreak is an outlier."

"An outlier?"

"Yeah. Someone who doesn’t fit the normal pattern – they are at risk, and you think they should’ve gotten ill, but didn’t.”

“What do you mean?”

“You remember the classic case study of the church picnic? Six hours after the picnic, all but one person who attended is vomiting. That person is your outlier. If you can figure out what was different about that one person, you might be able to solve the outbreak. Maybe he’s the only one that didn’t eat the tainted potato salad. So, you’ll have to ask around and find out what people may have been exposed to."

"Okay, Martinnnnnezz,” Bill said. “I'll be looking for that outlier. I can always count on you to give me a proper lecture. Thanks. I owe you one."

"No problemo. I only wish I could come up there and help you. Seems like I’m mostly buried in paperwork these days. Nothing beats getting my boots dirty again with some real investigative field work."

"Okay. Maybe we’ll figure out a way."

"Sounds good,” Martinez said. “Take care and let me know what you find."

"Right. Thanks, pal." Bill started to hang up the phone.

"Hey, Bill,” Martinez said. Bill put the phone back to his ear. “If you can’t reach me by phone, because I’m in a meeting or something, just e-mail me. Sometimes that’s more effective.”

Bill jotted down Martinez’s e-mail address.

"Ok,” Bill said. Let’s try to get together the next time I’m in DC. So long."

Bill hung up the phone and put Martinez’s contact information in his wallet. He took out the sheet of paper from his pocket with the list of diseases on it and copied some notes from his conversation with Martinez before replacing it back in his pocket.

The telephone rang.

"Bill?" Laura's voice was an unexpected surprise.

"Hi, Laura. Hey, I just got off the phone with my old Army buddy, Martinez. He's a public health doc. How are things at home?"

"That's why I called. Something's up with your dad."

Bill sat upright and sighed. "Is he okay?" he asked, apprehensively.

"He's more than okay, he's wonderful! You wouldn't believe it. He actually came out of his room this morning after you left and demanded a complete breakfast. He's really trying hard to communicate. His right hand's too weak to grasp a pen still, so he's working with his left hand. Unfortunately, I can't really decipher his writing, and he doesn't seem to want to type on the computer, but with practice and some help, he may do okay."

"That's amazing," Bill said, as he pounded his hand on the desk with excitement.

"That's just the beginning," Laura said. "He dragged me back to his study and pointed to some books on his bookshelf that he wanted me to get for him. I just peeked in there. He's got textbooks and articles strewn all about the room that he's reading."

"That's great" said Bill. "Just let him do whatever he wants. I don't want to hinder whatever's going on. I still have to make some phone calls, but I should be home in an hour or so."

"Great" said Laura. "I'll see you when you get here."

Bill hung up the phone, surprised at how elated he felt. Maybe his father would recover after all. He whistled as he leafed through the phone book for Mrs. Whitman's number. The phone rang again. "Yes?" he answered, thinking it was Laura calling back.

"Hello? I'm trying to reach Dr. Denton," a male voice asked.

"This is Dr. Denton."

"Dr. Denton, this is Dr. Rapaport from Saranac. We met last night in the ICU. I called to give you the sad news that Felicia Jamison has died. I'm sorry."

Bill gritted his teeth in frustration and put his hand over his eyes. He massaged his temples as Felicia's pustule-covered face filled his mind. Despite how ill she was, he still hoped she had a chance to recover. For a moment, he couldn't speak.

"Dr. Denton? Are you still there?"

"Yes, uh, sorry. I - I'm very sorry to hear that. I was really hoping she'd pull through. What happened?"

"She became progressively unresponsive with more difficulty breathing. She continued to deteriorate despite putting her on the ventilator. About an hour later her heart rate dropped precipitously and then she went asystolic. We coded her for over an hour, but it was no use."

"What did you list as the cause of death?"

"Varicella pneumonia. Her labs didn't have any big surprises: low platelets, acidotic – nothing unusual for someone with a severe viral pneumonia, but as you suggested, I *did* shotgun numerous other labs. I'll call you if anything unusual comes back."

"Thanks for letting me know," Bill said. "Are her parents there?"

"Yes – you want to speak with them?"

"Yeah, but it's probably not a good time. I'll try and contact them at home later."

"I'm sorry, Dr. Denton," Dr. Rapaport said. "We tried our best."

"I'm sure you did. Thank you."

Bill put down the phone slowly and sat for a moment without moving. He felt numb. He'd never lost two children so quickly before.

"Damn!" he called out and threw the phone book against the wall. It collapsed in a pile of bent pages on the floor.

He leaned forward with his head in his hands to absorb the weight of the news. He clenched and unclenched his fists in anger. How could he let this happen? He had to figure out what was going on.

The sound of children laughing startled him. He swiveled his chair around toward the window. A group of kids were playing ball in the neighboring field. "Could *they* be next?" he wondered.

15

African masks mocked Alfred Denton from the walls of his study as he sifted through his latest textbooks and articles. The faces, with rounded red mouths and wide black eyes, conveyed both surprise and fear, two emotions Alfred was feeling currently. Small ebony statues littered various end tables and bookshelves throughout the room. A large malachite pyramid served as a paperweight at the corner of his desk.

Alfred had overheard discussions between Bill and Laura in the kitchen the past few nights. The description he heard of Jeremy Whitman's illness jogged deep memories of his Peace Corps work in Africa over 30 years ago, when he had treated patients dying from some of the most terrible diseases on earth, like African sleeping sickness, malaria, cholera, and leprosy. Based on Bill's description of Jeremy's condition, Alfred knew that he'd seen patients with the same symptoms in the past, but the stroke had affected parts of his long-term memory. His struggle to remember the name of the disease tormented him. Meanwhile, the masks continued to stare at him as he could still hear the cries of children from decades earlier.

Alfred knew that Bill was a dedicated physician, but he hadn't experienced the type of medical conditions that Alfred had, in a place like Africa, with its rare, exotic diseases mixed in with the more typical types of diseases found in the United States. The challenge was figuring out when the disease was something routine and when to consider something more unusual. If Alfred could fit the diagnostic clues together that he overheard, he could alert Bill and Laura. He searched through page after page of his textbooks to find something to jog his memory. Whatever was out there could already be spreading, so he worked quickly.

Early in the morning, he ignored a slight tickle in the

back of his throat. As the day progressed, he felt occasional cramps in his lower back and thighs and some aching in his joints. Nonetheless, his drive to recall the name of the disease compelled him to dismiss them as stiffness from inactivity, so he continued reading intently, desperately searching for a diagnosis.

Bill eventually turned away from the office window. He pulled up a spreadsheet on the computer and typed *Case List* at the top, followed by a list of items:

Name
Age
Sex
School Grade
School
Address
Prior chickenpox vaccination?
Number of household members
Ill contacts
Symptoms
Vital Signs
Physical exam findings
Pertinent laboratories
Date of symptom onset
Date of rash onset
Date of death

Making two separate columns, he typed in the names of Jeremy Whitman and Felicia Jamison. Based on what he already knew, he filled out as much of the table as he could. After reviewing the information, he crafted a broad case definition to start with, as suggested by Martinez, which included any patient with a fever and a rash. The high fever lasted approximately two days. Death occurred in the two children about twenty-four to forty-eight hours from time of onset of the rash. The length of time for this disease to occur and worsen could be much longer, though, since these two cases might only be the worst ones. After all, with a disease like polio, for every person who ended up paralyzed, 99 others could have either less severe disease or no disease manifestations at all. He clicked on the print icon.

Bill picked up the crumpled phone book from the floor and looked up the Whitmans' address. After scribbling it on a slip of paper, he grabbed the spreadsheet and rushed out of the office. Cirrus clouds floated like white feathers painted across the sky's crisp, blue background, but the bright sun made Bill squint. He drove down Main Street past the Town Hall, grocery store, Post Office, pharmacy, and hardware store. The town was quiet with only a few pedestrians, which was typical for a Sunday afternoon. Ladies with bright orange and pink hats milled outside the local church where the service had just let out.

The bridgeboards clattered as Bill drove over the Bouquet River bridge on his way out of town. At this point, the river was at least 30 feet across. Foamy white water flowed between still, deep pools that probably were filled with trout. A couple bare-chested teenage boys sat in the middle of the river on a homemade raft of wooden planks lashed together with rope. They used their homemade fishing poles to cast their lines and bait into the river, hoping for a nibble. The scene reminded him of a similar adventure he had as a child floating down this very same river on a homemade raft.

About a half mile out of town, Bill turned down a narrow dirt road and drove about 100 feet before pulling up next to a small white trailer. The grass around the trailer probably hadn't been cut since the spring thaw and tickled his pant legs as he walked up to the door. After a couple knocks, Mrs. Whitman appeared.

"Dr. Denton?" she said, appearing surprised to see him. She had residual streaks on her cheeks and reddened eyes from crying.

"Hello, Mrs. Whitman. I am so sorry to bother you, but I really need to talk to you."

"Okay. Come in."

Upon entering the house, Bill noticed an earthy odor, like the smell of peat moss. He followed her into the living room, where the odor seemed to abate. The decorations were simple, with a light brown carpet, brown and gold striped curtains, and a matching faux leather easy chair and couch.

"Please sit down," she said.

"How have you been?" Bill asked as he sat down.

She rubbed her forehead nervously. "As well as can be expected, I guess. I haven't been able to reach my husband."

"Oh? I'm sorry. He's still in Washington, D.C.?"

"Yes - with our daughter, Michelle," she said. Tears glistened at the corner of her eyes. "He went along as a chaperone for Michelle's eighth grade class trip. They visit all the usual sights, so they're away from the hotel quite a bit. I've left several messages for him to call me, but I haven't heard a word."

"I'm sure he'll call as soon as he can, but if you need any help, I can get the Red Cross involved."

"That's not necessary," she said, her voice quivering. "I expect I'll hear from him soon."

"Would you mind if I asked you a few questions?" Bill asked.

"Doctor, I'm very sorry, but I really don't feel like talking." She pulled a tissue out of her pocket and dabbed her eyes. "It won't bring Jeremy back."

"Mrs. Whitman, I understand why you might feel that way." Bill leaned forward and softened his voice. "I promise it won't take long."

"Really, Doctor, I--"

"Mrs. Whitman," Bill spoke more firmly, but he hoped to hide the desperation in his voice. "Another child died this morning with something that appears very similar to what Jeremy had. I really, really need your help. Please. I'm very worried this could be just the beginning. You might have some information that could prevent more children from getting sick, and maybe more deaths."

"Oh," she said and then blew her nose. "Okay. I didn't realize--"

"It's okay. I should have mentioned it earlier. The other child's name was Felicia Jamison. Do you recognize that name? She was eight."

"No, but we've only lived here about six months."

Bill picked up a picture frame from the end table next to his chair. The photograph inside was taken at the beach, with Mrs. Whitman, Jeremy, a girl who appeared older than Jeremy, and a man.

"Who else lives here with you?"

"Just my husband, Michelle, and Jeremy – same as in that photo." She began crying at the mention of Jeremy. Bill set the frame down and pulled out his *Case List* sheet and a pen. He waited for her to calm down before asking another question.

"How old are you?"

"35."

"And the others?"

"My husband's 34 and Michelle is 13."

Bill jotted down some notes. "Did Jeremy ever mention any of his friends being ill recently?"

"Only Tommy Johnson, but you already knew that."

"That's right. Is it possible that Jeremy played with the Jamison girl without your knowledge?"

"Only if they had recess together, but that's doubtful. If she's eight, she's probably in third grade. Jeremy is…was only a first grader. After first grade, the kids move to a different building with a separate playground."

"Do you work?"

"Yes. I'm a housewife," she said somewhat

defensively.

"Of course. I understand," Bill said sympathetically. "What kind of work does your husband do?"

"I don't understand what use any of these questions have," Mrs. Whitman said angrily as she pulled out another tissue.

"I'm trying to find things you might have in common with the Jamison family, where a virus could have spread between the two of them, that's all. I don't know yet what might be an important connection."

"Oh." She calmed down. "Lately he's been working on a construction project."

"Has he mentioned anyone ill at work? Or has either of you been ill?"

"No."

"Has anyone else in the family ever had chickenpox?"

"Michelle and I had them for sure," she said as she counted on her fingers. "I don't know about my husband, but he didn't get sick when Michelle had it."

"Do you remember anything else about Jeremy's illness that might be important?"

"No."

Bill noticed a small brown mask hanging on the wall above the couch. It was highlighted with red and yellow streaks along the cheeks and forehead.

"Is that a ceremonial African mask?" he asked.

"Yes," she answered. "My parents were missionaries. I grew up in Africa. How did you recognize it?"

"My dad worked for the Peace Corps in Africa. He has a bunch of artwork from his travels strewn about his house. Perhaps you two should meet some day."

She didn't answer.

Bill got up to leave.

"Thank you for your help, Mrs. Whitman. If you think of anything else that might be useful, or if there's anything I can do for you, please call me any time." He gave her his cell phone number.

As Bill walked to the door, the earthy odor became more noticeable again. A pair of mud-spattered boots lay on the floor next to a mud-streaked doormat. Bill suspected they were the origin of the odor. He sidestepped the mat and departed.

Back at the office, Bill called the hospital in Saranac Lake and was able to catch Felicia Jamison's mother this time. She was naturally distraught, but willing to talk to him, nonetheless. He filled in Felicia's missing information on his *Case List* sheet. Mrs. Jamison and her husband were both 38 and also had a ten-year-old daughter. Mr. Jamison worked in construction, and Mrs. Jamison worked in the local liquor store. The parents had chickenpox as children, but the ten-year-old daughter had the chickenpox vaccine.

Bill compared the information from the two families. At first glance, two things looked interesting. First, Felicia Jamison's sister had been vaccinated against chickenpox, but she hadn't become ill. This should not be surprising, given the number of kids vaccinated every year, but he wondered if there was a reason Felicia became ill, but not her sister. Could the severe disease be related to when the person received the vaccine? Could there be a reason that none of the parents or siblings in the families hadn't become ill yet?

The second finding was that both fathers did construction work. Could there be a link? If they'd been infected on the job, it would be unusual for their kids to get a disease if the fathers never did. However, there were many diseases, like whooping cough, which might not make an adult very ill, but could be deadly in children.

He made a note to remind himself of those two potential clues so he could pursue them later. He recalled telling Laura he'd be home soon, so he put together some reading materials to take with him. As he walked out into the reception area, through the front window he recognized the mayor approaching the building. Bill took a deep breath before opening the door.

"Well, Sir, good to see you."

"Afternoon, Doc," the mayor barked, while chewing on a cigar like a piece of jerky.

"How can I help you, Henry? Are you looking for your sister, Rosemary? She's not working today."

"No. I need a word with you."

"Come in then," Bill said. The mayor walked past Bill before he could even gesture for the mayor to come in.

Bill caught a heavy whiff of cigar smoke mixed with whiskey as the mayor lumbered past him. Henry O'Donnell was in his early sixties. It had been at least a decade since they'd seen each other, and it was evident that the years had not been kind to him. His puffy face and body were covered with coarse skin and ape-like hair – very different from his sister, Rosemary.

"I haven't seen your pop since his stroke. How's he doing?"

"Making some progress, but you may not have heard, he suffered a second, more debilitating stroke. I doubt he'll ever work again."

"Shit. No, I hadn't heard. That's a damn shame. He's a good man. This town *really* needs him. I appreciate your stepping in to help out for a while."

"It's the least I could do."

The mayor had never really shown much appreciation for his dad, despite Alfred's many years of selfless service to the town. However, Henry seemed unusually cordial today - perhaps because Rosemary worked for Bill for the time being.

"Come into the office." Bill walked back through the clinic, followed by the mayor.

Bill gestured toward the chair opposite his desk as he sat down and leaned back against the bookshelf. He studied Henry, as he would any of his patients and couldn't help but notice his heavy breathing. Henry's obesity would make him a prime candidate for diabetes, hypertension, and heart disease, but Henry had never come to see him as a patient.

"So, Henry, I know you're too busy for social calls. Are you feeling okay? I assume you received my message?"

"Yes. It didn't say much, but I've heard about Jeremy Whitman and Felicia Jamison. What's going on?"

"How did you hear about them?"

"Everyone in this town knows everybody else's business, Doc. Rosemary told me about Jeremy, and someone in the post office told me about Felicia. I happen to know both of their parents."

"So, the word's out?" Bill asked.

"Not quite. I catch wind of *some* things that not everyone's privy to yet, but it won't take long 'til pretty near everyone will know - maybe in a day or two. When the kids go back to school tomorrow, word will run through this town like VD in a whorehouse.

Bill knew how quickly the panic level could spin out of control. Martinez warned him to make the media and the local government his friend. Henry could play a big part in quashing any rumors and disseminating appropriate information.

"The two kids died from what looks like severe chickenpox."

Henry ran his hand through his hair a couple times and frowned as he digested the information.

"Isn't that odd?"

"Yes and no…"

"Don't give me that crap!" Henry snapped. "I need answers."

Bill quickly remembered why else he disliked Henry so much. He always wanted things his way and only his way.

"If you'll let me finish, Henry," Bill said, holding up his hand, "I'll explain." Henry rolled his eyes and sat back in his chair. "Kids die of chickenpox every year but having two kids die within a day of each other in a small town like this is worrisome, to say the least. The way Jeremy died, with massive bleeding, is particularly concerning – I've never seen it before with chickenpox, although I know it can happen."

"Is this thing contagious?" Henry's hands made sickening bone crunching noises as he cracked his knuckles.

"If it's chickenpox, then it's very contagious, but it's generally mild, and most people are already immune to it. You know that. I'm sure you had it as a kid, just like me. When it kills them, though, there's usually something wrong with their immune system, rather than from the virus itself. Usually if someone's going to die from chickenpox, they're older or pregnant."

"What are you doing to check this out? By this time tomorrow, I'm going to be bombarded with phone calls from every concerned grandmother, mom, dad, aunt, uncle, and third cousin twice removed from here to Albany."

Bill sensed Henry's fear, like a presence in the room that oozed from Henry's skin. His fat lips pursed tightly as he clenched his jaw. It was hard enough to understand medical risks as a physician, but even harder to explain risks of disease to non-medical people. Bill was the mayor's lead medical authority in town, so he needed to help him out of this potential public relations disaster.

"Henry, I'm happy to talk to anyone you want me to. Sometimes people like to hear things from a doc. So far, I haven't found much that these kids had in common. I've sent a bunch of blood specimens to the lab to identify an organism, but those will take some time –"

"How much time?"

"A couple days at least, maybe as long as a week or two."

"What? Goddamn it!" Henry smacked the desk. "Do we have that kind of time?"

"At this stage, your guess is as good as mine. I don't know if this will turn into something bigger. Are these the only two cases we'll see? I don't know yet. If this is chickenpox, most people should be immune, so it shouldn't spread."

"What can we do *now*? I'm not talking next week here."

"I've already left a message for the school principal. If this thing escalates, the school's the first place this will spread, and we might need to close the school or limit public gatherings. Those measures could help interrupt transmission, but things would have to become pretty drastic to do that."

Henry clearly wasn't pleased by this information. He grunted as he got up from his chair with some effort and started pacing back and forth in front of the desk. The sound of his heavy footsteps on the wooden floor echoed throughout the entire clinic.

"It may be helpful to put something in the local paper to alert people," Bill said. "I'm concerned, though, about blowing the whistle too early. If these two cases end up being the last ones, we'll get slammed for jumping the gun."

The mayor stopped pacing and shook a finger at Bill.

"That's for me to worry about," he said.

Henry moved to the window next to Bill. The orange hue from the setting sun glowed on his puffy face.

"Doc," he said in a low voice, his jowls shaking, "I've lived here my entire life. I love this town. We thrived when I was a kid when the Adirondacks were the playground for the rich city folk and a haven for tuberculosis victims. When airplanes became the big deal, this place became a forgotten welfare wasteland. All those rich folk hightailed it to places like Aspen or Vail. Who wants to take a train to the Adirondacks to ski on the icy slopes of Whiteface, if they get all the powder they want out west? Who gives a shit about swimming in an Adirondack lake when it's just a hop and a skip to Hawaii? Folks here don't take pride in themselves no more. They sit around lollygagging on their porches waiting for a government handout."

Henry's voice nearly cracked a couple times as if he

might cry. Bill was moved by his raw emotion. He even began to feel pity for Henry. Had he misjudged him? Tears glistened in Henry's eyes from the setting sun.

"You see," Henry continued, "you were lucky. Your father had enough money to give you a ticket out."

Bill nearly interrupted Henry to remind him that the Army funded his schooling.

"I never had that luxury." The corner of Henry's mouth tightened, and his voice turned coarse and angry. "My father skipped out on us and left us nothing. It took years for me to support ma and rebuild what we had."

Bill shifted uncomfortably. Henry's words provided great insight into his mindset.

"Doc," the mayor said, still gazing out the window. "I'm going to make up for all the years we've been crapped on. I have a dream for the Adirondacks...for this town. This town will be reborn. To hell with government handouts! The resort we're building on Glacier Lake is the *key* to that rebirth."

Henry swerved suddenly toward Bill and grabbed both arms of his chair. He stuck his face so close that pores on his nose looked as large as nail holes. The burned-out cigar nearly touched Bill's cheek. Henry's voice was quiet and firm, and his laser-like eyes pierced through Bill.

"These deaths are a problem, Doc," Henry said with foul cigar and whiskey breath. "Any bad press could fuck up my project. Don't you *dare* talk to the press."

"But Henry," Bill protested, his muscles tightening and his anger building. "Rumors are going to start flying. You can't stop them."

"You let me worry about that. I'll decide when we talk to the local press. We've got to work as a team. We can't afford to make a false step. You call me if you get any new information and if there is anything I can do to help you stop this disease. You're the one with the fancy medical degree. Figure out what's going on and STOP IT...but do it quietly.

The press must be a measure of last resort! They'll take something small and spin it into a crisis for no good reason."

Henry paused and turned again toward the window. Only then did Bill realize he was holding his breath.

"Got it, Doc?"

Bill couldn't take it anymore.

"No. I don't *got* it."

Bill held up his index finger and waved it as a warning toward Henry's face.

"I'll follow your plan only so far," Bill said. "We're on the same side here. I'll keep you informed, but I'll do whatever it takes to protect the people in this town. That's *my* job. If that means going to the press, then I'll do it, no matter what you say."

Henry seemed caught off guard by Bill's response that he wasn't easily intimidated. He appeared to struggle with how to respond.

"Uh, yeah, good" Henry mumbled. "Now, if you find out anything important, you give me a ring right quick. Good night."

Henry turned abruptly and left the room. His footsteps echoed all the way to the outside door. The door opened and slammed shut, followed by footsteps fading away in the distance.

Bill sat there for a moment, still boiling. Henry O'Donnell was a classic bully, and he wasn't going to let him dictate medical policy. As with any bully, once he stood up to him, he backed down quickly.

Darkness crept into the room as the sun slipped behind Cobble Hill. Bill paced the room, remembering Henry's burning eyes. Was Henry really concerned about the town's future or just his own profit motive?

Bill picked up the paper on his desk and could barely read the words *Case List* in the faded light.

"Bastard!" Bill said aloud, resolving to protect his patients at all costs.

He put the case list in his pocket and called Norm Phinney's number at the morgue, but there was no answer. He resolved to visit Norm first thing in the morning to see if he'd found anything useful from his autopsy of Jeremy Whitman. Then he threw some papers and patient files into his briefcase and headed for the door.

16

Norm stirred Alfredo sauce into a pot of tortellini and removed it from the stove. He placed a small amount of water into a saucepan with fresh cut asparagus and turned the burner on high. Until today, his legs had felt like rubber, but now he'd finally recovered both his strength and his usual voracious appetite. The scab on his finger had contracted down to the size of a pencil eraser and would probably fall off in a few days.

He chopped up some garlic, which sizzled as it landed in another saucepan with melted butter. The aroma of the garlic made his mouth water and his stomach growl. His excellent culinary skills had fostered his already large girth over the past several years. Despite having limited funds to repair a leaky roof and repaint his run-down house, Norm never skimped on his food, even when others teased him about his weight.

The phone rang. Norm maneuvered slowly to the phone around a half-full bucket of water in the middle of the kitchen, which he used to catch rainwater.

"Hello?" Norm answered.

"Dr. Phinney?"

"Yes?" Norm thought the voice sounded familiar but couldn't place it.

"This is Dr. Thompson, from Keene Valley."

"Oh yes." Norm now recognized the voice – a family practice doc from the neighboring valley. "What's up?"

"I wanted to let you know about a patient I'm sending you."

Norm had a queasy feeling. Dr. Thompson sent a fair amount of laboratory samples and would occasionally send him a stiff when he needed an autopsy.

"Tell me about the patient," Norm said.

"He is – I mean was - an 18-year-old construction

worker. His boss brought him in yesterday – looked like severe chickenpox. He was really sick."

Norm suddenly became much more interested.

"Chickenpox?"

"Yeah. I tried to transfer him to Saranac Lake last night, but all their intensive care beds were full, so I kept him here overnight. It was hell! He bled massively in the middle of the night. Damned if I've ever seen anybody die like that."

"What did he look like?" Norm momentarily imagined the pale face of Jeremy Whitman lying in the morgue.

"Like a goddamn monster by the time it was all over. I CODED him for over an hour, but he didn't have a chance."

"Have you contacted the family?"

"No – don't know how to reach 'em, and I haven't had a chance to call his boss who brought him in."

"You want me to hold him, then, until you reach the family?" Norm asked.

"Sure. I'll see what I can do. I'd *love* to know what killed this guy. I've never seen chickenpox kill anyone. Can it do something like that?"

"I think so, but not often," said Norm, feeling fear building in his gut.

"I requested an ambulance about 15 minutes ago. The body should reach you in about 45 minutes. Sorry about the short notice."

"Yeah, well I *would* appreciate some more notice in the future."

Norm had trouble hiding the irritation in his voice. He contemplated chewing out the doctor but then thought better of it. After all, it was a small community. He should be thankful for the referral. Besides, he needed to determine whether the features on this body matched those of the Whitman boy.

"Ok. I'll head into the hospital soon," Norm said, "and I'll be there in time to meet the body. My assistant is out this week. I'll let you know what I think after my external exam. If he died within 24 hours of entering your facility, it's a medical examiner's case."

Norm considered telling the doctor about Jeremy Whitman's death but then decided to wait. He could never be sure what to expect until he actually saw the body, since the descriptions of corpses on the phone didn't always live up to reality. If there was no similarity at all, he didn't want to spread any false information.

"I'll keep trying to reach the family," Dr. Thompson said. "Thanks."

"Sure," said Norm skeptically as he hung up the phone.

He caught a whiff of something burning and noticed smoke rising from the stove across the room. "Damn!" he yelled as he stumbled into the rain bucket, knocking it over and drenching the floor. Norm cursed himself for not emptying the water after the last storm. He splashed his way to the other side of the room and yanked the pan off the burner, nearly burning his hand in the process. He swore as he dumped the crisp black asparagus into the garbage.

Putting his food disappointments aside, Norm couldn't help but feel some rare excitement but also foreboding. This was the rare case that required a trip into the office on a Sunday. If this man looked anything like the Whitman boy, chickenpox or no chickenpox, he would declare it a medical examiner case. The last thing he wanted to do was rush his dinner, so he poured the tortellini into a plastic container and placed it in the fridge. He threw together a large sandwich, grabbed a soda, then left the house and drove to the hospital, completely forgetting about the soaked kitchen floor.

17

Bill locked the office door and stepped out into the dark evening. The Milky Way spanned the length of the moonless sky while a few fireflies danced about the grass, intermittently flashing like dying meteors. An occasional dog bark broke through the usual buzz of crickets chirping. As Bill unlocked the car door, the sound of his cell phone ringing startled him. He recognized the number at the morgue.

"Hi Norm," Bill said, "I called you earlier, but you weren't around. Anything new on Jeremy Whitman?"

"I got some lab results back, but that's not why I called you. You need to come here and take a look at something."

"What's up?" Bill asked, his interest rising.

"I'll explain when you get here."

"Okay. I was just getting in my car. See you in a few."

Bill made the short drive to the hospital in less than five minutes, passing through the center of town on the way. For a small town, the government buildings were quite impressive – large red brick structures with slate roofs sprawled across several well-manicured acres of grass. At this hour, the windows were nearly all black, except for a few lonely office lights. Bill wondered whether Henry O'Donnell was back in his office. The rest of the town was empty except for a few teenagers milling around the youth activity center. He remembered doing the exact same thing when he was their age. Most of the friends he used to hang with peaked as varsity athletes in high school and hadn't gone real far since. He ran into them periodically at the grocery store. A couple of them were on welfare, another worked for the highway patrol, and one had died in a mining accident. Henry O'Donnell was right in one regard: Bill's father's influence on him had given Bill incentive to strive for something beyond the town. The place hadn't changed much since he was a kid – a new grocery store and pharmacy, but otherwise, the town seemed locked in a previous era.

Bill parked in the back of the hospital and made his way through the basement catacombs to the morgue. Norm looked a little disheveled and lacked his usual grin.

"Hey Norm, what's bothering you?"

"I could use a little food, but more importantly, we've got some bad shit. Come over here."

The tone of Norm's voice made Bill feel uneasy. He followed Norm reluctantly over to the wall with a bank of four stainless steel refrigerator doors, feeling increasing alarm.

"I'm starting to fill up in here," Norm said.

Norm yanked on some gloves before pulling open the second drawer and jerking the sheet down. "Here's our chickenpox victim." Norm gestured toward the cadaver.

Bill recognized Jeremy Whitman, with scattered darkened purple pools under the skin left over from where he'd bled, in sharp contrast to his otherwise uniformly gray skin. Much of the blood had settled toward his back from gravity, called livor mortis. In addition, small circular bumps punctuated his face and arms where the vesicles had been. The bumps had a different character now, flatter and wrinkled, like deflated balloons. In fact, their appearance now seemed very familiar.

"Sorry to bother you, Jeremy," Norm said sarcastically. "So, Bill, I called you because of my latest package that arrived from Keene Valley today."

Norm moved over to the third refrigerator drawer and pulled it open. A yank on the sheet revealed a man who was probably in his late teens and freshly dead. Bill stared aghast at the corpse. His skin was pale and ashen, but horribly disfigured and peppered with pus-filled boils all over his body. Many of the pustules had coalesced to form even larger pockets, like water droplets that run together. Several large bruises surrounded the larger pockets.

"He's a monster," Bill said. "You couldn't dream up

something this horrible, even for a horror movie."

The pattern of lesions looked exactly like those of Jeremy Whitman *and* Felicia Jamison, with more on the face and hands than on the chest. Bill took a deep breath and closed his eyes tightly, wishing this all might just disappear. He leaned against the wall, crushed by the weight of the evidence. Whatever this was, it was spreading.

"His name is Scott Guernsey," Norm said, "an eighteen-year-old construction worker from Keene Valley." Norm tore off his gloves, chucked them in a red biohazard wastebasket, washed his hands, and then grabbed a yellow hospital file off his desk. "I got some of his medical history from the doc in Keene Valley, but there's more information in his chart. His illness started two to three days ago with a high fever. A day later the fever subsided, but he developed skin vesicles. Last night he called his boss...a Mr. Jed Thorton, who took him to Keene Valley Hospital. Once there, he had a rapid decline in his mental status and massive hemorrhaging."

Bill's mind again filled with visions of Jeremy Whitman the night he CODED in the hospital.

"If I had to bet money," said Norm, as he closed the patient chart, "I'd bet he's got the same thing as Jeremy, our friend behind freezer door number two."

"Yeah, I kinda figured that."

Bill then informed Norm about Felicia Jamison. "Felicia was a little different than these others. She didn't bleed like them, but the pattern of her rash was the same. I wasn't sure until this point, Norm, but now there's no doubt: this is an outbreak. What could *do* this?"

"Do you still think it's chickenpox?" Norm asked. "I mean, three kids in twenty-four hours dropping like flies?"

"No way! This can't be chickenpox without some other factor involved. Did this guy get the chickenpox vaccine?"

"I doubt it. How long's the vaccine been out?"

"Only a couple years. You've got his records there. Let's look."

The two of them found the yellow international shot card stapled inside the records. The edges of the card were frayed and the writing smeared in places.

"Let's see," said Bill, as he leafed through the shot card, "cholera - no, yellow fever - no. Here are the miscellaneous listings: oral polio 1, 2, 3, and 4, Diphtheria-Tetanus-Pertussis 1, 2, 3, 4, and a tetanus booster last year. Measles-Mumps-Rubella once at 12 months old and a booster when he went to high school. That's all that's on here. No chickenpox vaccine. I guess that blows my theory."

"What theory was that?"

Bill explained his concerns that the vaccine against chickenpox might have had something to do with the severe illnesses. “If this Guernsey fella wasn't vaccinated, then my theory is shot. There *must* be something else going on."

"Either that, or he received the vaccine, but it was never documented in his chart."

"Yeah, but as you said already, he’s probably too old to have gotten it anyway, and I wouldn’t be surprised if he had it as a kid."

"Could those kids have anything else in common?"

Bill thought for a moment. He pulled out the case list from his pocket.

"You know, there *was* one other thing. Both parents worked in construction. Didn't you say this guy was a construction worker?"

"Yeah. I wrote down his boss’s number, in case you wanted to call him." Norm rifled through the numerous stacks of papers and computer parts cluttering his desk. "Here." He handed Bill a yellow slip of paper with a phone number scribbled on it.

Bill recognized the area code for Keene Valley. He grabbed the phone and dialed.

"Thorton here," a gruff voice barked on the other end.

"Mr. Thorton, this is Dr. Denton. I work over in Elizabethtown and I -"

"Hey Doc. Are you that young fella from Washin'ton that took over for your old man?"

Bill winced at being called *young*. "Well, yes, that's me. I'm helping out…for now."

"I tell you, son, your daddy's a heck of a doc. I don't think I'd be here right now without him. D'ya think I could come see ya sometime--"

"Sure thing. Just call and make an appointment, but sir, I called because I need to ask you some questions about your worker, Mr...uh" - he read the name on the chart – "Scott Guernsey. You brought him to the clinic in Keene Valley last night?"

"Yeah. Poor guy. Looked like a nightmare. What's he got?"

"I'm trying to figure that out, Sir. I don't know if you've heard yet, but he died today."

There was a pause on the phone.

"Holy crap! No! Not Scott! Son of a bitch! Son...of...a...bitch! What happened?"

"His doctor thinks he died of chickenpox." Bill waited a moment to let some of his news sink in. "Mr. Thorton?"

"Jed. Call me Jed."

"Okay, Jed. Do you know if Scott's been around any children lately?"

"Hmm. He was a good boy, that Scott. He and the other boys stayed out at the worksite most o' the week. They've got kids, but not Scott. He ain't got no family here. On weekends, he goes into Keene Valley to hit the bars, but I doubt he's seen any kids.

"What kind of construction are you doing?"

"Construction? Ha! If it keeps up like this, I'll be in the poorhouse soon!"

"I'm sorry, Jed, I don't understand."

“I've got a contract to lay some drainage and sewer pipe and some site excavation before they put in the foundation. We haven’t done squat for two days. At this rate, I'll lose the job. One of my boys skipped off to Washin'ton. Next, Scott calls in sick. Shit, today, Jamison says his kid's–”

“Jamison?” Bill asked. “Did you say Jamison?”

“Yeah. His girl’s sick, so he runs off to Saranac Lake. I don't know what the hell's goin' on, but I can't lay pipe by myself."

Bill became very excited. "Jed, do you have another worker named Whitman?"

"Hell yeah, and I've got a mind to fire his ass, skippin’ off to Washin'ton like that."

Bill saw the puzzle pieces falling into place.

"Sir, where have you been laying pipe?"

"Up the side of Glacier Lake – buildin’ a big hotel."

Bill opened his eyes wide. "Jed, did you find a dead body up there a couple weeks ago?"

Norm’s eyes popped wide open.

"Damn straight,” Jed said, “about two weeks ago. Socked into the ice, he was."

"Do you remember who was with you that day?"

"What day?"

"The day you found the body."

"Oh. Well, let's see. It was me and all my boys: Otis Whitman, Roger Jamison, and Scott Gurnsey."

"Who found the body?"

"Hmm, Scott spotted it first from the backhoe. The frozen dude’s hand was stickin’ out of the trench."

"Then what happened?"

Jed explained how they’d all pitched in to remove the body from the ice.

“Was anyone wearing gloves?" Bill asked.

"We all wear work gloves, but that bastard was so slipp'ry, I think we took ‘em off just to keep a hold on 'im. Say, what's all this about, anyway? Have I done somethin' wrong?"

Bill measured his words before answering. "No sir, I'm just trying to get some information. You see, your workers, Mr. Whitman and Mr. Jamison, each have a child who died in the past two days, and now Scott Guernsey is dead." There was silence on the line. "Jed, are you still there?"

"Doc. Am I in danger or somethin'?"

Bill's mouth felt dry. Jed definitely had a risk of infection with whatever the others had, especially if it wasn't chickenpox - - but it was looking less and less like chickenpox. "I'm going to be straight with you, but I also don't want to make you paranoid. So far, it appears that the victims have been young, but I really don't know what we're dealing with. There's a strong possibility you've been exposed to something. That's why I'm going to have to keep a close eye on you. How do you feel?"

"Ok. Why?"

"You don't feel sick in any way? Have you had any fevers?"

"No...well, I *have* been a little tired and felt a little warm the last couple days. My eyes and throat were a little sore - - but it was no big deal, Doc."

"Any bumps on your skin?"

"Maybe a couple pimples, but nothin' unusual."

"You're sure?"

"Yeah."

"Nothing like what you saw on Scott Gurnsey?"

"Hell no, thank God!"

"And you're feeling okay now?"

"Yeah."

"Sir, did you ever have chickenpox?"

"I think so - my momma said I did."

"What about your family members? Are they okay?"

"Just me and the wife. We're both good."

"How old are you and your wife?"

"I'm 55 and she's uh...how old are you Mabel?" Bill heard Jed's wife scold him through the muffled receiver. "The missus is 49."

"Sir, if you haven't gotten ill yet, there may be a reason. If these children died from chickenpox, you're probably not at risk. If you start to feel sick, especially if you get a fever, call me immediately. Regardless, promise me you'll come by my office tomorrow morning so I can examine you." He gave Jed his number.

"Doc, if my boys' families are in trouble, I want to help them. What can I do?"

"I don't think there's anything you could've done to prevent this, Sir," Bill said, "but I'm sure your worker's families would appreciate your support now."

"Ya know, Doc. I'm a retired Army sergeant major. I take care of my own. I'll go ask their wives if I can help them out."

"I'm sure they would appreciate that. Would you prefer I call you Sergeant Major?"

"Nah, that's okay. I gave up the title long ago. Were you in the military?"

"Yeah, Army also – hooah - - ten years. I left when I was a major." Bill and Jed exchanged some stories of their overseas deployments. Jed had gotten out just a couple years ago - the same as Bill.

"Thank you for your time, Jed. Don't forget to come see me."

"Yeah."

Bill hung up the phone. Norm's eyes surveyed him with anticipation.

"We've hit it, Norm!"

"Hit what?"

"The jackpot!"

"What do you mean?" Norm asked

"The body, Norm, the body."

"Which one?" Norm shrugged his shoulders and

gestured toward the cadavers on the other side of the room. “Drawer number two or three?”

"Neither, you turkey! Don't you see?"

Norm still shrugged his shoulders and shook his head, appearing frustrated with Bill’s guessing game.

"Sorry. I guess you couldn't hear what Jed Thorton said.” Bill repeated what he’d learned. “That frozen body might be the key to this whole outbreak. Do you still have it?"

"Yea, drawer number 1, next to Carol Merrill. Do you want to trade it for the prize behind the curtain?”

“Very funny, Norm.”

“Don’t worry. I’m still trying to identify that stiff, so he’s still mine. I’ve been so sick lately that I haven't been extremely motivated, either."

Bill snapped on some gloves and went over to drawer number one and pulled it out. He yanked down the sheet.

“Damn! Check this out.”

"What?" asked Norm, as he moved in next to Bill.

“Compare the lesions on John Doe here and those on Jeremy Whitman. You can imagine that they could eventually look almost exactly alike. Scott Guernsey’s are more prominent, but still similar.”

“You’re right,” said Norm. “I *thought* something was familiar about it. The pattern is the same on the face and extremities. Shit! I can’t believe it!”

“What?”

“Remember what I told you a couple weeks ago - - how it looked like there was bleeding under the skin around the lesions? I can’t believe I didn’t connect that to the same findings I saw on Jeremy Whitman. I just never considered the two could be linked."

“Neither did I,” said Bill, “until now. Have you gotten any lab results back on John Doe?”

Norm informed Bill about the contaminated bacterial cultures and the virus culture that was still undetermined.

“My God!” Bill swore. “Could this body have carried

something alive? Damn! I can't believe it. This is like some horror movie where an Egyptian mummy is unearthed and unleashes some scourge."

"Only we don't know if there will be a happy ending," Norm said.

"Exactly." Bill grabbed the handle of one of the freezer doors. "Let's put these guys back on ice so we can figure out our next move."

Norm joined him and the two of them pulled the sheets on the bodies back up and then closed the drawers. Bill tore off his gloves and threw them into a red biohazard bag. Norm did the same, but his hands were shaking. They both washed their hands.

"So, what now?" Norm's voice betrayed his nervousness.

"We need to figure out what it is, but wait-" he snapped his fingers -"that's probably not as important as determining how it spreads. You and I went through our medical training around when HIV first surfaced. Remember? Even before they ever isolated an organism, they pinpointed the spread through sexual contact and the blood supply. By acting quickly, they saved countless lives. We need to do the same." Bill hurried across the room and grabbed a magic marker from the whiteboard behind Norm's desk.

"Do you remember when they unearthed the body?" Bill spoke as he wrote furiously on the board.

"You kidding? Hold on. Let me check." Norm sifted through some papers on his desk. "Here it is: May fourth."

Bill wrote the date on the whiteboard. "Today is May 20th. Jeremy Whitman's symptoms began two days ago and he died yesterday. Felicia and Scott had similar time courses."

He scribbled a chart quickly:

Day 0, Body found: May 4

Jeremy Whitman – Symptoms began D+14, May 18, died on May 19

Felicia Jamison – Symptoms began D+14, May 18, died on

May 20
Scott Guernsey – Symptoms began D+13, May 17, died on May 20

Bill stepped away from the whiteboard and reviewed what he'd written.

"If we assume Scott Guernsey was exposed on the day the body was found, then the incubation period would be somewhere around two weeks. The two children wouldn't have been exposed directly to the body, but their fathers were. If this disease is contagious, how could it jump to the children, but not affect the fathers? That doesn't make any sense. If the parents didn't get ill, then they shouldn't be able to transmit the disease to the kids. Perhaps they *did* catch it, but it affects kids worse than adults?"

Norm nodded his head in agreement. "Maybe. Or maybe the parents are immune to it somehow?"

"That's possible, I suppose, but how?" Bill leaned up against the desk and dug his knuckles into his forehead. Surely, he could figure this thing out. It had to follow the usual patterns of disease spread. "I think we're making some progress, but we've still got some key issues." He held up his hand and counted on his fingers. "First - how could the children get infected without direct exposure to the body? Second - why aren't Mr. Jamison and Mr. Whitman sick, or for that matter, Jed Thorton, or any of the workers' wives? Jed Thorton probably had the most exposure when he face-planted right into the hand. If we can figure out those issues, we can crack this thing."

"One thing you've overlooked, Sherlock." Norm picked nervously at his fingernails.

"Oh yeah? What?"

"The second wave."

"What do you mean?"

"If this thing is really contagious, then our time is running out...fast. What about all the people exposed to these victims already? I'm not talking about a frozen organism that's been dormant for God knows how many years and probably weakened over all that time. I'm talking about fresh, hungry, deadly pathogens that have just finished partying in a warm body and have jumped onto a new host, primed to reproduce, like in *Alien*. I'm talking about *you*, Bill." Norm emphasized his point by poking his finger into Bill's chest. "You were breathed on by Jeremy Whitman *and* Felicia Jamison in the last day or two, at the peak of their infections. Their bodies were probably teeming with organisms. I'm talking about *me too*! Son of a *bitch*!" Norm collapsed onto a stool as the weight of this realization knocked him down. "I got stuck with a dirty scalpel from that fucking corpse!" Norm rubbed the scab on his pinky as if trying to rub it off. "I'm talking about *anyone else* around those patients – and that includes the hospital staff and the other family members." Norm's voice trembled. "How long do we have until our faces start exploding with pustules or we bleed like stuck pigs? Two weeks? Or less?"

18

Otis Whitman tried to ignore his aching neck muscles all morning, but as the day progressed, the throbbing pain spread to his lower back and thighs. He rubbed his neck hoping it would reduce the pain, but he felt extremely cold and shivered. The odor of rubbing alcohol in the clinic brought back unhappy memories of receiving childhood shots. The clinic's exam room was quiet, except for Michelle's hacking cough and an occasional word from the doctor who examined her.

Otis already explained to the doctor the progression of Michelle's sickness, starting with a headache on the flight down to Washington, D.C. A high fever started suddenly the next day during their Capitol and White House tours. Despite his insistence that she rest in the hotel, she refused to miss the opportunity to tour the nation's capital with her classmates, even though she looked like hell. This morning, though, Michelle became worse. They accompanied the class to the Smithsonian Air and Space museum and watched a movie on the history of aviation. As the movie presented Charles Lindbergh's trans-Atlantic flight, Otis noticed Michelle sweating heavily next to him and she began to cough nonstop. When the lights came on after the movie, Michelle had tiny pimples all over her face and she was breathing fast. He took her immediately to the nearest medical facility.

He made numerous unsuccessful attempts to call his wife and cursed himself for never buying an answering machine at home. They hadn't spoken since the trip started. The doctor's bright red hair and freckled face made him appear younger than Otis would expect for a doctor. He bent his tall, lanky body awkwardly over the exam table as he assessed Michelle. Various diplomas covered the walls: a BA from Princeton and an M.D. from Duke. Otis wished he'd pursued more education. He'd gotten married and the children arrived before he turned 22, making it more imperative to find work than to go back to school.

The doctor finished his exam and hung his stethoscope around his neck. His voice brought Otis back into the present.

"Mr. Whitman, I need to speak with you, please."

The doctor gestured toward the door. Michelle gave him a worried look through bloodshot eyes. Hair on her arms glistened with tiny beads of sweat and wet strands of hair stuck to her face. The white sheet of paper covering the exam table was soaked and clear from Michelle's sweat. The tiny pimples he first noticed on her face had multiplied and grown in size, with larger bumps now appearing on her arms and legs.

It must not be good, Otis suspected, otherwise the doctor would share the information in front of Michelle. Her deathly green skin tone scared him. She'd never looked this sick before, even when she had pneumonia in third grade. Otis' headache intensified as he stood up. A searing pain crept up the back of his neck and down his back.

"Uh…everything's going to be okay, sweetie," Otis managed to stammer, as he feebly attempted to give Michelle a reassuring smile.

"We'll be right back, Michelle," the doctor said as he opened the door for Otis. "Everything's going to be fine."

The doctor closed the door and followed Otis out into the hall. He moved in very close and spoke in a low voice.

"Mr. Whitman, I don't want to alarm you, but I need to level with you." The doctor suddenly didn't seem so young. "Your daughter is very ill. I think she has a very severe case of chickenpox, including pneumonia, although it's too early in the time course of the rash to be sure. Has she ever had chickenpox?"

"I don't know. My wife probably would."

"I need to admit Michelle to the hospital immediately."

Otis tried to swallow, but his mouth felt too dry. He knew the doctor was right, but he didn't want to accept it. A bill flashed in his mind - a very expensive bill that he knew he couldn't afford.

"Uh, isn't there some medicine you can give her? I...I don't have very good health insurance." He closed his eyes and dug his knuckles into his temples, as the pounding in his head became unbearable.

"Right now, we need to get her into the hospital, and we can worry later about how her bill is paid. She needs immediate treatment. Her temperature is 104 degrees. Her blood pressure is low, and she's breathing fast. She might already have what we call varicella pneumonia, which is very dangerous. I'm going to admit her directly to the intensive care unit."

"Uh, okay. I just want her to get better. What do I tell my wife?"

"Let's get Michelle plugged in over at the hospital first. Then I'll be happy to explain everything to your wife."

Otis' hands shook. The hallway started spinning and dark shadows closed in on his peripheral vision. His legs gave way, and he fell back against the wall for support. He could no longer understand the muffled words coming from the doctor. *This is not good*, he thought, trying to shake off the aching in his shoulders and back muscles. Lancing pain shot from the base of his skull to his tailbone. A sudden chill made him shiver uncontrollably. *This is not good at all.*

The doctor's eyes bored through him as Otis slid helplessly down the wall, unable to muster the energy to hold himself up or cry for help. Sweat mixed with tears trickled down his face.

"Mr. Whitman, are you okay? Mr. Whitman? Nurse! Come here STAT!"

19

Laura picked up the ringing phone. She was surprised by the voice on the other end. “I couldn’t reach Dr. Denton at the office, so I thought I might be able to reach him at home,” Mrs. Whitman said amid gasps and sobs. Her daughter, Michelle, was gravely ill in the intensive care unit in a Washington, DC hospital, along with her husband, although he wasn’t as sick as Michelle. Both of them were covered with boils, and none of the doctors knew what was wrong with them. They were considering chickenpox, typhoid fever or Rocky Mountain spotted fever. Mrs. Whitman was leaving for Washington, DC immediately.

After Laura hung up with Mrs. Whitman, she phoned Bill’s office. There was no answer, so she called his cell phone. No answer. A little while later, he called back from the morgue and assured her he’d call the hospital in Washington, DC immediately.

Laura put down the phone and poured herself some coffee. In the still kitchen, the clicking of the wall clock seemed amplified. It was already 10:00 pm. She had hoped Bill would return before nightfall, but she was accustomed, *too* accustomed, to the time demands of a doctor's life. She reminisced about her ex-fiancé, a surgical intern, who she dated in nursing school. His long hours in the hospital gradually eroded their relationship. One night she planned to surprise him on his birthday while he was on call. She brought him dinner to his call room and found him in bed with another woman. After that, she vowed never to get involved with another doctor. The anger and hurt seemed to have finally subsided, as she began to feel close to Bill. Was it a mistake?

Not wanting to second-guess fate, she pushed those thoughts aside. This job gave her flexibility and a decent income. Bill was fun to be around, so why close any doors prematurely?

As the cool night air crept like a sinister presence along the kitchen floor, the warm coffee mug felt soothing and made up for the lack of a warm fire. She set the mug down on the kitchen table and re-opened the book she'd been reading before Mrs. Whitman's call. The book, about the discovery of vaccines, read more like a medical mystery than a history text, as she went back in time to stories about whole civilizations decimated by dreaded scourges like plague, smallpox, and cholera. Some day she hoped to teach medical history, so she cracked open her notebook and began to scribble notes. As a wide-eyed girl with pigtails, her grandfather had filled her with tales of plague-infected fleas being dispersed over Chinese cities during World War II. The creative ways humans found to destroy one another never ceased to amaze her.

As she flipped through the pages of the 1800s and 1900s, the book begged her to read more, but her eyelids became heavy. She reluctantly gave in and closed the book and left the kitchen. The hallway was dark, except for a sliver of light on the floor coming from Alfred's partially opened bedroom door. An hour ago, he indicated he wouldn't need her assistance for bed, so she tiptoed quietly past his room. The stairs creaked as she climbed past remnants of Alfred's African travel. In the dim light, a bright blue and orange tapestry hanging from the banister had transformed to brown and gray. A five-foot-long spear clung to wall by the stairwell.

When Laura reached the upstairs bathroom and turned on the light, she appraised herself in the mirror. Her straight black hair barely caressed her shoulders, and her bangs hung just above pencil-thin eyebrows. She wished they were bushier so she wouldn't have to highlight them each morning. A few gray hairs had cropped up recently, and she was losing in the battle to pluck them out as more seemed to appear. Her sharp cheekbones were still smooth, but small creases began at the corner of her eyes. She used a gentle cleanser to wash off small amounts of eye shadow and mascara.

As she left the bathroom and turned off the light, rays of light filtered in through the bedroom window from the porch outside, casting shadows from the trees against the wall. She flicked on her room light. The bedsprings of the large mahogany poster bed creaked as she sat on the edge and slid out of her white knit top and blue jeans. She folded each article of clothing in turn and piled them neatly on her bedside chair. Her eyes were naturally drawn to the full-length mirror in the corner of the room. Her breasts were ample for such a petite woman, and her stomach and leg muscles remained tight and trim from her regular exercises. One noticeable feature was a large scar on her left upper thigh, about the size of a quarter. She never knew the cause, other than it occurred around the time of a trip to Taiwan when she was three. Children used to tease her about it in the summer, which to this day, made her reluctant to wear a high-cut bikini. For many years, it retained a reddish tinge, which made it more easily visible, but more recently the color had faded to a hue that was closer to the rest of her skin. She unconsciously rubbed her thigh, as if to erase the scar, feeling its uneven surface. Turning away, she threw on a nightshirt, then pulled down the white comforter and hopped into bed. The springs creaked as she bounced up and down momentarily while getting into a comfortable sleeping position. After switching off the light, she hugged her down pillow in the darkness. The red glow of the digital alarm clock persisted in her mind even after her eyes had closed and she drifted off to sleep.

Alfred Denton spent the evening searching frantically through his medical library. Despite his efforts, he still couldn't find anything in his new textbooks that was compatible with what he'd overheard Bill and Laura discussing. After his fruitless search, he began to doubt himself.

The aching in his joints that began in the morning progressed to his lower back. His skin began to feel like someone stuck him with thousands of tiny needles, but he ignored the pain, intent on pursuing a diagnosis. The light outside had long since faded and he had heard Laura go upstairs. It was time to call it quits. He slammed the textbook shut and massaged his pounding temples.

As he lifted his head, he noticed a small ebony statue that he'd purchased in Africa on the edge of his desk. It had stood there for years, so most days he barely noticed it. It was no more than four inches tall but was heavy enough to use as a paperweight. It cost him a pretty penny, because the superstitious Africans used it to ward off a scourge.

He grunted as he strained to get up from the desk, and his head pounding intensified. His paralyzed arm ached so he massaged it with his good hand. He felt a bump under his fingers and looked down at his arm. Oh. It was only his smallpox scar. *Smallpox. Smallpox. What was it about that name?* On a whim, he picked up the ebony statue and examined it closely. The face was contorted painfully, and it had the disfiguring pockmarks typically left behind by the disease. *Smallpox*. That's why it cost him so much. Smallpox was ravaging Africa when he worked there. The eyes had a blank stare, symbolic of the cruelty of the disease and its ability to cause blindness.

"No!" he grunted aloud. The statue slipped out of his hand as a wave of memories flooded his mind. The stench of rotting, sloughing flesh hung like fog in the air of the infected villages where he worked. He saw children in thatched huts gasping for breath with their skin covered head to toe by horrible pockets of pus. Those were the lucky ones. They had a chance to recover, but they were left with lifelong scars, bone and joint deformities, or blindness. Others didn't live beyond a few days and bled from every orifice – their crimson eyes searing through him from their deathbeds.

The statue splintered as it crashed onto the wooden floor. Now he knew why Bill's description of the dead children seemed so familiar. He'd stepped over dozens of similar decaying carcasses decades ago. He fell back down into the chair with a thud. *Could it be? Could smallpox, the most horrific disease ever known have returned?!* It killed more people on earth than all of the wars combined. He didn't want to believe it. He couldn't believe it.

Alfred frantically lunged for his textbook again and tore through the pages to find smallpox, as his head felt like it would explode. There was only a half page in the book on it, stating that it was declared eradicated in 1980 by the World Health Organization. Only two places in the world still kept the smallpox virus frozen in storage: the CDC in Atlanta and the Vektor labs in Russia. The planned destruction of the virus stocks had still not happened, as the global public health leaders repeatedly pushed back the dates.

He flipped through some of his other new textbooks. No wonder he hadn't found anything - none of the newer books had more than just a passing mention of the disease. It had been forgotten. He pulled an outdated textbook from the bookshelf, copyrighted in 1980. A quick search in the index revealed a complete chapter on smallpox. He nearly tore the pages in his haste to find the chapter. The image of a distressed child with the most horrible, disfiguring rash stared at him from the page. The child had so many large pustules on his face that many had joined together, essentially turning the child's face into one large pocket of pus. Alfred was convinced - this had to be the disease that afflicted Bill's patients.

Alfred remembered how difficult it had been for him to believe that smallpox had really been eradicated. The last time it surfaced in the U.S. was 1949, but his intimate knowledge from dealing with hundreds of victims in Africa made him skeptical that it had really gone for good. Without any viable treatments, prevention was the only solution. So, he saved a vial of the freeze-dried vaccine in his office freezer – just in case the World Health Organization had made a mistake. It had been a long time since he'd checked on it. Now, with his head pounding, and his memory uncertain, he couldn't be sure it was still there. Did he throw it out?

The implications of what he'd just discovered overwhelmed him. The aching in his leg, neck, and back muscles crescendoed. His skin burned as if he'd been hit with a blowtorch and sweat gushed out of him. The sudden and severe onset of his symptoms puzzled and scared him. He hadn't felt this bad since he came down with malaria. A sudden nausea overcame him, and he hobbled into the bathroom barely in time to vomit. When he was done, he splashed water on his face, trying to rid himself of his headache and his terrible discovery. In the bathroom mirror, he didn't recognize the face that stared back at him. It was too old, unshaven, reddened from a likely fever, and now he noticed small pimples covering it. Each one seemed to have a deep origin and burned as though he'd been touched with a lighted cigarette. He looked down at his arms and hands. Similar small pimples had blossomed there as well.

"No!" he stammered, suddenly recognizing his own demise.

His bare feet slipped on his own sweat, and he lost his balance. His chin came crashing down on the sink, before his body fell backwards. His head cracked against the toilet, and he heard a loud snap as severe pain shot up from his right hip. He lay on the floor for minutes, gritting his teeth to fight the pain. His right foot was rotated outward – that hip had surely fractured.

Blood from his chin smelled like raw meat as it oozed onto his chest and then the floor. The tempo of his throbbing head accelerated – he estimated his pulse must be around 140. He tried to scream for Laura, but he could only muster a weak "La."

How could he have gotten smallpox? How was he

infected? It didn't make any sense.

He felt a deep, vice-like pressure in his chest, which made him hyperventilate. He clutched his chest as the crushing began to suffocate him.

I've got to tell Bill. He grabbed the doorframe with his good hand and managed to pull his body sideways. He slid over the floor on a mixture of blood and sweat out into the bedroom, with the searing pain in his hip causing him to grunt with even the slightest movement. Images of the room blurred and darkened. As he lost consciousness, the pain in his hip and chin subsided, and a cool, calming sense of euphoria enveloped him. He wondered again whether he might have saved some vaccine.

Laura awoke with a sudden jerk. Had she been dreaming or did she really hear a loud bang inside the house? She sat up in the darkness and strained to listen but only heard the occasional creaks of the house and crickets humming outside. The digital clock's red numbers glowed 11:00.

The floor creaked as she stepped on some loose boards on the way to the door. She paused to listen again but only heard the wind rustling the pine trees outside. A small amount of light still shone into the downstairs hall from Alfred's room, which struck her as odd at this late hour. She put on her robe and grabbed a brass candlestick to use as a weapon, just in case. With deliberate hesitation after each step to listen for an intruder, she slowly made her way downstairs.

20

Bill hung up the phone after talking with Laura. The possibility of a new wave of cases frightened him, especially with the news that Otis and Michelle Whitman were sick in Washington, DC. He washed his hands three times with an antiseptic solution, as if somehow that could wash away the unfolding outbreak.

Bill said, “Up to this point, Norm, I hadn’t seriously considered my own risk, but you’re right. Not only could we become victims, but so could anyone else who had contact with the first cases. Do you think it’s possible that your illness after you cut your finger could’ve been a mild form of this disease? If so, then maybe you’re already immune.”

“That’s wishful thinking,” Norm said, holding up his pinky, “but my scab didn’t look anything like the rash on those patients. I still think my finger was a garden-variety *Staph* infection like you thought before. Besides, it got better with antibiotics.”

“Maybe,” said Bill. He wasn’t completely convinced the antibiotics did anything, but he decided not to burst Norm’s bubble.

“It’s pretty much gone,” Norm said, “except I’m stuck with an ugly scar.”

“You should be glad that’s all you’re stuck with,” Bill said. "Okay, buddy, let’s focus on a plan of action.” He picked up the marker again. He described to Norm the steps Martinez had suggested for investigating an outbreak: make a case definition, make a list of cases, and then identify common aspects of the different cases. Finally, look for an outlier.

He wrote *fever and rash* on the board as his case definition. “In order to count cases, we’ve got to find them. Let’s alert all the hospitals or clinics around these parts to be on the lookout for patients who meet that case definition.” He wrote down on the white board *1) alert hospitals.*

"I don't have any doubt now where the initial exposures occurred," Bill said, "so we need to target the affected families, put them under observation, and feed them information as we learn it."

He scribbled down the names of all the construction workers and their family members, and put an asterisk next to anyone who was already ill or dead:

Mr. Jed Thorton
Mrs. Thorton
**Mr. Otis Whitman – in Washington, DC*
Mrs. Whitman
**Michelle Whitman – in Washington, DC*
**Jeremy Whitman - dead*
**Scott Guernsey - dead*
Mr. Roger Jamison
Mrs. Jamison
**Felicia Jamison - dead*

"So, we have three dead so far and two currently ill. Next, we need to alert the press."

He wrote *2) Call the newspaper.*

"How about the mayor?" asked Norm.

"Right. I already spoke with that bastard."

"What gives?" Norm asked. "Why so negative?"

Bill described his run-in with Henry in the office and his concerns about the mayor's motives.

"I see your point. Why not forget about him then?" Norm asked.

"I'd like to," Bill said, "but Henry could play a key role in helping us avoid a panic." He wrote *3) Keep mayor informed* on the board. "Do you have your cell phone on you?"

"Yeah," Norm said.

"Great. You call the surroundings hospitals in Keene Valley, Lake Placid, and Saranac Lake."

"Hold your horses, dude," Norm said, holding up his

hands. "The only cases we have so far are two construction workers, and three immediate family members. We don't even know how this thing spreads, yet. What am I supposed to tell these hospitals? Are we going to cause panic for no reason? Maybe it won't go beyond the families."

"Maybe, but with three dead already, I'm not going to sit on my hands waiting for the grim reaper to drop more bodies like wasps sprayed with RAID. Each of those hospitals handled one of the patients, so their employees and maybe even other patients are at risk. The least we can do is alert them to determine who had contact with the patients and put those people under observation. Every hospital has an infection control nurse. Tell them the case definition and what we've seen already. Let them hunt down any of their staff and patients who may have been exposed and monitor them for a fever.

"I get it. So, if the people who worked on the patients *do* get sick, what do we do with them?"

"Treat them - *if* there is a treatment. So far, we haven't been too successful, but at least we'll know who is sick and needs to be monitored or treated and we can get them out of circulation to stop the spread. We also need to target anyone else they may have been in contact with. Damn! The number of people under observation could multiply exponentially. I'm calling the county health department again now." Bill punched the numbers on his cell phone with one hand and scribbled *4) Call county health department* on the white board with the other. Bill pointed the marker at Norm. "Get dialing, Norm."

"Yes, sir!" Norm gave Bill a mock salute.

Bill also wanted to get in touch with the Washington, DC hospital to see if they had any additional ideas about what was going on. He held his phone to his ear and wrote *5) Call Washington hospital*.

Norm began phoning while Bill first called the health department. No one was there again, but he left a message for the director to call him as soon as possible. He did the same for the town newspaper. Next, he called the mayor at home.

"O'Donnell here," a groggy sounding voice answered.

"Henry, this is Bill Denton."

"What? What's going on? What time is it?"

"About 11:30." Bill updated him on the situation and what he wanted to do.

"Doc, you're out of line. It's my job to declare a crisis. So, you linked all those people to the construction site? Big deal! You've got nothing that proves it's gone beyond that. I can help you put them under observation, but that's all you need to do now."

"You're wrong," Bill said. "I'm sitting in the morgue with two new stiffs already. Another one's dead in Saranac. Three dead, Henry! And two in intensive care in Washington, DC. How many more do you need?"

Bill tapped his fingers on the lab bench in anticipation of Henry's answer.

"We can still handle this within our community."

"What are you talking about?" Bill asked, feeling his face flush with anger. Henry had never seen how quickly meningitis could move through a college dorm or how resistant *Staph* bacteria could contaminate a hospital. He just didn't understand how quickly a disease could lead to a disaster.

"This is *already* outside the community, Henry. We need to do something…and fast."

"You cocky son of a bitch. Let me handle this. You city boys think you know it all. I know a thing or two about dealing with a crisis. We can keep a lid on it."

"That's bullshit!" Bill yelled, his anger popping like a champagne cork. "Get your head out of your ass! If you don't listen to me, your whole fucking town and your precious Adirondack dream are going to be buried! If you really care about this town, you'll shut your ass up! I'll fly straight over your head like an F-14 and bring in the governor if I have to."

Bill paused. Had he pushed too hard? Were there really more victims out there waiting to spike a fever? He couldn't be sure. If he was wrong, the mayor could legitimately ride his ass out of town. The other end of the line was silent.

"Henry?" Bill said quietly.

"I hear you, loud and clear," Henry bellowed. "Perhaps I was rather abrupt." His gruff tone became conciliatory.

Bill silently tapped the lab bench in triumph – he'd stood up to a bully and won.

"Listen," Henry continued, "I'm very concerned about this situation, too, but we need to be extremely cautious on how we handle it. If you start an uproar, there's no telling what'll happen next. I don't know how much time we have before something leaks out of Washington, DC, but I'd guess two days or so. We can still be the first to present it and put the right spin on this, okay?"

Bill hesitated, but he was willing to go along with it as long as he could do what he felt was appropriate in the meantime.

"Okay," Bill answered.

"I'll alert the other mayors around here. We can handle this. I'll have the sheriff send his boys out to the construction workers' homes to reassure them. There's no doubt they'll get wind of this and get panicky."

"Don't worry," Bill said. "I'm going to contact all of them as soon as I hang up."

"Good. First thing in the morning, we'll talk with Rodney at the paper together."

"Great. I'll call you tomorrow. Out here."

Bill hung up. Norm was still talking on his cell, so Bill called the Thortons and the Jamisons to alert them that the sheriff might drop by. There was no answer at the Whitman home. He dialed the Washington, DC hospital numbers Laura had given him. He was able to reach Dr. Wortmann, one of the infectious disease docs working in the ICU there who updated him on the patients.

"Michelle Whitman is now on a ventilator," Dr. Wortmann said, "and she's starting to bleed from various body sites."

"What do you think is going on?" Bill asked.

"Our working diagnosis for her was initially severe varicella pneumonia, but once she began bleeding, we've had significant internal debate whether this could be Rocky Mountain spotted fever, typhoid fever, or a viral hemorrhagic fever, like Ebola or Marburg. Some of the docs have nearly come to blows. To be candid, though, none of our diagnoses thus far have panned out, and we're baffled."

"Wow," Bill said, "that makes me feel a little better that I'm not the only one. How is Michelle's father doing?"

"He has a more significant rash, but a milder illness overall without any bleeding or breathing difficulty." Bill then described the other cases that occurred in Elizabethtown.

"Let's stay in touch," Bill said, as he hung up. Norm was just finishing his call. Things seemed to be working out. Bill triumphantly informed Norm about his conversation with the mayor, and the doctor in D.C. Norm's tight jaw and thin lips belied his discontent.

"What's the matter?" Bill asked.

"I just had the receptionist in our emergency room on the line," Norm said in a shaky voice. "She said the ambulance just rolled in with your dad."

"What?"

Just then Bill's cell phone rang. It was the ER calling.

21

May 20, Midnight (D+16)

Bill parked in the back of the hospital, then ran down the dark basement hall and took the stairs two at a time to the first floor. Laura met him in the ER. She explained the state she found Alfred in.

"He's been unresponsive for over an hour, since I found him," she explained to Bill.

"Ok. Thanks." Bill joined the ER team and took control of the CODE for another half-hour before reluctantly calling it off. It was a position he could never have imagined he'd be in – running a CODE on his father and then, like the hand of God, having to throw in the towel and pronouncing him dead. He was surprised how rapidly things unfolded, but it wasn't unusual that a stroke patient would die of a massive heart attack.

After he ended the CODE, Bill collapsed on a chair in the corner of the room, as he felt the weight of what had just transpired. Laura guided him to the quiet room to give him some time to process what happened. She stayed with him while the nurses cleaned Alfred's room. Bill barely recognized the nurses, technicians, and hospital administrative personnel who paraded through the quiet room to express their condolences, even though he'd known some of them for years. He felt Laura's comforting arm around his shoulders as she fended off the various visitors.

"No," Laura said to the charge nurse, "Dr. Denton does not want an autopsy."

Bill found himself numbly nodding in agreement. After the visitors left, he sat, staring at the floor, his mind a blur, as Laura consoled him. Eventually he regained his composure and was ready to leave.

"Laura," he said, "I don't know how I could've

handled this without you."

Laura gave him a warm smile and comforting hug in response.

There was a quiet knock on the door, followed by the chief nurse sticking her head into the room.

"Dr. Denton? The room's clean now. You can go and visit with your father."

"Thanks," Bill said.

Laura held his arm as they walked to the room, past the stares and whispers of the hospital and emergency room personnel.

The odor of sweat and blood in the room had been replaced with the scent of rubbing alcohol and bleach. Only a dim fluorescent light illuminated the head of the bed. Alfred's ashen face poked out from beneath the white sheet that covered him from the neck down; his expression was one of quiet calm. Alfred's sudden death did little to resolve their differences, but Alfred seemed at peace, which helped to quell Bill's growing anger and sadness. Alfred's battle was over. As Bill approached the bed, some contrast cast by the light accentuated something on Alfred's face that caught his attention.

"Laura" – he gripped her hand and pulled her away from the bed - "do you see that?"

"What?" Laura had a puzzled expression. "Are you sure you're up for this?"

"Yes, but look." Bill flicked on an auxiliary room light. "Damn! I didn't notice it during the heat of the CODE, but look at his skin," he said, pointing at Alfred's face. "See these tiny fluid-filled vesicles?"

"Oh, my God!" Laura let go of Bill's hand and covered her mouth. "I uh…everything happened in such a rush, and it was dark in the ambulance. I…I didn't notice them either."

Bill pulled on a pair of exam gloves and yanked down the sheet.

"They're on his hands too. See?"

He tore off his gloves and threw them into a red biohazard container. He bolted out of the room and down the hall to the nurse's station.

"Dr. Denton," the ER nurse asked, "is everything okay?"

"No," Bill said, slightly out of breath. "Listen up. I need you to call in the infection control nurse right now. Have her contact me STAT!"

Bill immediately called Norm and demanded that he do an autopsy on his father after all. Norm promised to complete it, along with the others, as soon as possible. The infection control nurse called, and Bill told her to add anyone who had contact with his father to the list she'd already started for contacts of Jeremy Whitman. Despite the late hour, she said she'd be right in and would also speak with the county health department in the morning.

Laura drove Bill's car for him while he called Henry O'Donnell. The mayor seemed a little more receptive this time.

When they got back to the house, Laura fired up the coffee maker while Bill jotted down some notes and ran the events of the past couple days in his mind, searching for clues.

"I don't understand it," Bill said. "Dad didn't leave this house for the last two weeks. The incubation period for this killer appears to be around two weeks. The only people he's had contact with are you and me."

Laura handed him a cup of coffee.

"And Nettie. Remember? She brought over that food?"

"Oh, yeah."

"But how could he have been exposed?" Laura asked. "There's no plausible connection between him and that frozen body or any of the construction workers."

Bill began to pace the room, wracking his brain for answers.

"He must've had contact with someone who was already transmitting this disease – but maybe they had a mild case and didn't even know they were infected. If it wasn't one of us then it must be Nettie. But if she's the one, I can't believe she wouldn't have gotten sick by now."

Bill called Nettie immediately. Despite being awakened, Nettie said she felt fine. While they were talking, Bill informed her about Alfred's death. Then he remembered something Nettie had said a couple weeks earlier.

"Nettie, the last time I saw you, you mentioned something about when you were a child, and the Sheriff made everyone stay in their houses. Do you remember any more about it since we spoke?"

"I'm sorry, Doc. It was a long time ago. My only recollection is it was sometime around 1946." Bill thanked her and hung up.

"So?" Laura asked.

"She feels fine, so I doubt she could've infected Dad. What about the possibility that he didn't contact the pathogen from a person? What about an object?"

"Like what?"

"The first time Norm showed me that frozen corpse in the morgue, when he yanked down the sheet, I had a strange feeling that something might have landed on me. Maybe even in my eye or on my clothes."

"Come on, Bill," Laura frowned, "that sounds pretty far-fetched. This whole night -- this outbreak -- has got to be overwhelming for you."

"Wait a minute," Bill protested. "I'm serious." He continued pacing while talking. "Hear me out. My dad being infected has enormous implications. If he was infected, then who else? I don't remember, but I'm sure I would've worn gloves the first night I looked at that corpse. But isn't it *possible* that something might have gotten onto my clothes? I think I leaned against the morgue table when I was examining the corpse's skin lesions. Maybe I brushed up against the body. If so, I could potentially spread it to someone else, right?"

"I guess – but it would have to be a pretty hardy organism to live outside the body. And then it would have to contact the other person in the right spot on the mouth, nose, or eyes."

"Exactly," Bill said. "It must be a hardy organism if it could survive on a dead body buried in the permafrost. Then you agree that it's theoretically possible?"

"Uh, yes…theoretically, I guess," Laura answered. "Would you stop pacing the floor? You're making me nervous."

"Sorry." Bill stopped pacing. "So maybe I'm not completely crazy. Do you remember the night I came home after seeing that body?"

"I'm not sure."

"That was the night Dad came in here while we were eating. He was all upset, and we had to sedate him."

Laura nodded.

"I jostled with him a bit to calm him down. Surely if I had something on my clothes, he could've had contact with it then. That could also explain why these construction workers' kids got sick about the same time as their parents. Maybe the kids gave them a hug when they got home - - dirty clothes and all."

"Well, I guess it's possible."

"Damn!" Bill banged the table, startling Laura. "How else could you explain it? When I visited Mrs. Whitman yesterday, there was this decaying smell in the house - like mud mixed with rotting vegetation. Sure enough, I noticed some muddy work boots by the door. If dad could be infected by my clothes, then why couldn't Mr. Whitman's kids get infected by their father's dirty boots or clothes?"

"Except you've ignored something, Laura said."

"What's that?"

"Why aren't *we* sick?"

"Yeah. I haven't ignored it, I just can't explain it. If I could, then I'd know how to stop the outbreak. Maybe we're immune somehow. Or maybe it's still growing inside us. There's one thing I have to assume now, but I couldn't be sure before. We've both been exposed. The *real* question is whether or not we'll get sick, and how long we have before that happens."

Laura sighed, her eyes glistening in the kitchen light. She had a sober expression on her face as she looked down at her hands. Bill walked over and gave her a hug.

"It'll be okay," he whispered in her ear and kissed her on the cheek.

She turned to face him and her tender, warm lips met his. They lingered together for a moment before she pulled away and wiped tears from her cheeks.

"This is too weird," she said. "I work for you. I'm supposed to be consoling you. Things are already complicated enough."

"You're right. I'm sorry," Bill said, stepping backward.

"Oh hell," Laura said, and she grabbed his waist and pulled him in for a tight hug. "Neither of us is ill, so we should just count our blessings. We can support each other through this."

"You're right," Bill responded, and he hugged her back. "We can lick this, whatever it is. The answer is there, if we just ask the right questions." He stroked her shiny black hair and gazed at her. "You know, you're even more beautiful when you're upset."

"Stop it. Don't embarrass me." She squeezed his arm. "By the way, what was that all about with Nettie on the phone - something about her childhood?"

"Oh – glad you asked." Bill became serious. "When I first told her about the frozen body a couple weeks ago, we got to talking about people getting lost in the hills and freezing to death. Apparently, when she was a kid, sometime around

1946, the whole town was locked down because of some guy from New York City."

"I don't understand," Laura said. "What could that have to do with what's going on now?" She grabbed a tissue and dabbed her eyes.

"I didn't make any connections at first either, but now I'm starting to wonder. What could be more frightening to a small town than an escaped convict - something so scary that the sheriff would lock down the town?"

Laura shrugged her shoulders.

"How about the Grim Reaper? Some terrible disease. Maybe the town was under emergency quarantine."

"I guess it's possible, but I can't imagine quarantining a whole town. It's not something we deal with anymore."

"Exactly – not anymore – but if Nettie's right about 1946, we're talking over 50 years ago. Things were different back then, and that's why I didn't think about it – until now."

22

May 21 (D+17)

Bill stepped over to the window facing the back yard. The kitchen light behind him cast his shadow a good twenty feet onto the ground outside. He couldn't see beyond the small rectangle of light that surrounded his shadow, but beyond that light he knew a green field stretched for a hundred yards before gradually sloping upward into a foothill and eventually blending in with towering Bald Peak. Bald Peak was just the first mountain in a series of mountains someone would have to climb, including Rocky Peak Ridge, and Giant Mountain, before they could reach Keene Valley on foot. He'd done the rigorous climb into the wilderness over the peaks and valleys as a teenager with friends. It took nearly 16 hours. Somewhere out there, beyond the mountains, children and their parents slept, unaware of what could eventually turn their towns into jails – possibly just like Elizabethtown sometime around 1946.

"Maybe there's a way we could track down what Nettie was talking about," Bill said. "If it was *so bad*, then there must have been something in the town paper about it."

"Okay," Laura said, "I'll go to the library first thing in the morning."

"Exactly, but I don't mean in the morning – I mean now."

"Are you crazy? It's way past midnight." Laura put her hand on his arm. "Don't you want to just take a break tonight?"

"Of course I do." Bill held her hand in both of his. "But I can't. *We* can't. This has been a horrible day, one of the worst days of my life, but I can't bring my dad back. Right now, I am more concerned about the living. This thing is moving too fast. We don't have any time to lose." He let go of her hand and stroked his chin. "Tell you what. I really need to search on the Internet and through my dad's books for an organism that could survive long enough to be transmitted by someone's clothes. Can you go to the library for me?"

"Of course." Laura frowned. "But how can I get in at this hour?"

"Not to worry." Bill lifted his right hand and patted her cheek. "It just so happens that the librarian, Mrs. Lillian Johnson, is one of my stubborn, but beloved patients. In fact, I saw her grandson, Tommy, with chickenpox just a couple weeks ago. It's about time for her usual follow-up appointment, so this can serve as a reminder. While you get ready, I'll call her and convince her how important this is."

"All right. Be back in a sec."

Laura left the kitchen and Bill phoned Mrs. Johnson. Sure enough, he'd awakened her. Once she overcame her initial shock and fear from receiving a call from her doctor at this late hour, she agreed to meet Laura at the library.

Bill hung up the phone just as Laura returned.

"Everything okay?"

"Perfect. She'll meet you there in about 15 minutes. Of course, she made me promise to give her a free office visit, and I could only oblige." They discussed exactly what Laura was looking for. "Make sure you call me the minute you find something - anything."

"Of course," Laura said. She leaned forward and gave him a peck on the cheek and then moved to the door.

"Hey," Bill called after her. "Thanks…for everything."

Before leaving, Laura turned and blew him a kiss.

In his father's bedroom, Bill was met by the stench of blood and sweat still lingering in the air. For the time being, he sprayed some bleach over the areas contaminated with blood, resolving to clean them thoroughly as soon as he had more time and after he'd exhausted his search for information. In the study, he grabbed his laptop and one of his dad's infectious disease textbooks from the bookshelf. He settled down at the kitchen table with a cup of coffee and searched the Internet and read the book intently, searching for the right organism.

The anthrax bacteria won the prize for an organism that could survive for decades outside the body in its spore form. If someone had a large amount of dry powdered anthrax spores on their clothes, it was conceivable that any close contacts might be infected, but the type of skin lesions that anthrax caused – usually single black scabs - didn't look anything like the numerous pustules on his patients. Norm Phinney's finger scab looked similar, but it wasn't black.

Typhus and relapsing fever were transmitted by lice, which lived in the linings of people's clothing. They could cause a rash as well as bleeding, but he hadn't noticed lice on any of the patients, and once again, the skin lesions looked very different. The pattern of spread also seemed to be too quick. He made a note of those diseases, but none really fit.

Bill pulled the case list he'd made from his pocket and reviewed it once again. He added his father's name to the list. By rereading the list, he hoped that something might suddenly appear obvious that would guide him on how to proceed next, but there was nothing. He reviewed his *to-do* list. Norm had already alerted the surrounding hospitals. Bill had a meeting in the morning with a journalist and the mayor at the town paper. The county health department hadn't called back yet, but he would try them again as soon as the office opened. The labs he'd sent on Jeremy Whitman hadn't come back yet, so he needed to check on them as well as the ones sent by the Saranac hospital on Felicia Jamison. By sun-up, they should have some bacterial culture results, although viral cultures could take several days. He rubbed his drooping, dry eyelids and attempted to fight the need for sleep, but he felt himself drifting off. As his mind faded off into oblivion, he wondered how Laura was faring. There really wasn't much more he could do until he heard from her, or until morning, so he gave in.

Laura sped down the valley road from New Russia to Elizabethtown. Despite a gnawing feeling in the pit of her stomach from worrying that she might have been infected, she couldn't help feeling excited helping Bill investigate the outbreak. This kind of fieldwork - researching historical clues - really appealed to her. The road to Elizabethtown was completely deserted, except for a fox she nearly hit as it darted out in front of her headlights. The town was dark and deathly quiet as she entered. Intermittent streetlamps, covered by swarms of moths, cast a light-yellow glow down Main Street. She drove past the grocery store and town hall before turning down a side street to the town library. The lights on the porch and inside were already on. Laura parked the car and walked up the squeaky wooden stairs. She smelled fresh paint on the white shingled building, which shimmered in the moonlight. Scattered drop cloths and paint cans indicated that the exterior work continued.

Laura knocked on the door, and a moment later, a thin woman with gray hair tied up in a bun greeted her. She wore a brown raincoat and sneakers, and she peered over wire-framed reading glasses with a scowl.

"Hello, Laura," she said in an unexpectedly pleasant voice, given her old school marm appearance. "I'm Lillian. Come in, come in." She waved Laura in.

"Thank you," Laura said. She entered and found the interior had a cozy feeling and resembled a hunting lodge. The knotty pine-paneled walls were adorned with deer and black bear trophies. Despite its small size, there were numerous computer terminals scattered throughout the main room between magazine racks and book stacks.

"Wow!" Laura said sincerely. "I love the look of this place!"

"Thank you, dear. My late husband was an avid hunter, and he donated the trophies. I've attempted to maintain the hunting lodge-themed decor. I figure if people feel comfortable, they're more likely to spend time here."

"Well, now that I've seen it, *I* certainly will come back again, but I'm sorry you had to come in tonight. I'm not sure how much Bill told you, but we've got a very serious situation, and we need your help."

"I know the basics: some large news event around 1946. Unfortunately, the library burned to the ground in 1950, so we don't have any original newspapers before then, but we were able to make microfiche from copies stored at the newspaper office for the 1930's to 1970. Come here, I'll show you."

Laura followed her to the far end of the room, where she pointed out the microfilm machine and a brown metal filing cabinet against the wall. Lillian pulled out a drawer near the middle and removed two small boxes.

"These two film reels contain the papers for 1946 and 1947. Until 1950, the paper only came out weekly, unless there was a special news bulletin. Do you know any more details about when this event occurred in 1946?"

"Unfortunately not. According to Nettie Baker, everyone in town was ordered to stay in their houses – something about an escaped convict, but Bill's concerned that it may have had something to do with that frozen body they found a couple weeks ago at Glacier Lake."

"Oh, yes. I heard about that," Lillian said, while looking at the two microfilm boxes. "It's hard to keep a secret around here, especially if Nettie hears about it. She knows everything." She handed Laura the box for 1946. "Looks like the *Elizabethtown Tribune* had 52 issues that year."

"Thanks," Laura said, as she threaded the film into the machine.

"I wish I knew what Nettie was talking about," Lillian said, "but 1946 is just a little before my time. A lot of the town cleared out just after the war to look for better economic opportunities, so there's not many others still around these parts who would've been old enough to remember something that happened in 1946 – perhaps old man Dillard up on Cobble Hill - but he's half deaf, and his mind's not what it used to be."

Laura scanned through the microfilm for information, hoping that if there were something of real concern, she'd find it on the front page. The machine whirred as she pushed the lever and successive pages flew by on the screen.

"You see," Laura said, "Bill is starting to suspect that this frozen body could be linked to recent deaths in town – that maybe the big scare in 1946 was *really* related to a disease outbreak and nothing to do with an escaped convict."

"My land!" Lillian exclaimed. "Wouldn't that be something? People are already talking about some of the kids. They're scared."

"Not surprising," Laura stated. "That's all the more reason we need to get to the bottom of this, quickly."

They reviewed the entire year together, one front page after another, but didn't find anything exciting – just the usual small-town events like the town board elections, the school prom; somebody bagged a large deer; and other news.

"Nothing useful here," Laura said. She rewound the film. "You also have 1947?"

"Yes."

"I guess it wouldn't hurt to check that as well."

"The label says there are 54 issues," Lillian remarked. "Maybe they had some special news bulletins that year."

"We'll see," Laura said, feeling her pulse quicken as she traded film boxes with Lillian.

She threaded the film onto the machine. The film hadn't been rewound since it was used last, so she began at the end of the year and worked backward, once again perusing the headlines. Laura's pulse quickened as she pulled up a special edition for April 1947. She scanned the headline.

“Well, this is probably what Nettie was talking about. She read the headline out loud. “Elizabethtown Hit With Storm of the Century. Despite the recent hints of an early spring, the Elizabethtown community was pummeled with a massive ice storm, which left the entire Adirondack region without power for over a week. Crews continue to try and re-establish power to remote sites. Local residents are advised to stay inside. Outdoor conditions and driving in the area continue to be extremely hazardous. Be wary of the risk of contact with live, fallen power lines.”

“Well,” said Laura. “There it is. It’s interesting how a young girl’s imagination can distort things.”

“You’re right about that,” Lillian replied. “Why don’t you at least print it out while you’ve got it?”

“Good idea – at least it might satisfy some of Bill’s curiosity.” Laura pushed the *PRINT* button. “I’m sorry I got you out of bed for this.”

“It’s okay, dear,” Lillian said. “I’m happy to help. Let me know if there’s more I can do – I am so sorry to learn about Alfred’s passing. He did a lot of good for this town, and now Bill has been a great resource in the short time he’s been standing in here. I hope he’ll stay.”

“So do I,” Laura said. She grabbed the printed page and got up from the chair. “By the way, do you have any Internet services?"

"Oh, yes. We have two computers that connect. I’m proud to say that we’re the only public facility in town that offers it. Newer technologies generally tend to come late to a small town like this, but we’ve recently installed a satellite link. Now we no longer have to worry about getting hooked up through the limited phone lines coming into town. You're welcome to sign up for an access account."

"Thanks, but it’s late, I don’t want to bother you with it now.”

“It’s no bother – after all, we’re both already wide awake. I won’t be able to get back to sleep anyway.”

"Okay. Thanks." Laura put down her newspaper copy, filled out the Internet form, and handed it to Lillian.

"And here's your password," said Lillian as she handed Laura a slip of paper.

Laura put the paper in her purse, and then she picked up the newspaper copy and glanced at it again. At the bottom of the page was a smaller article that she hadn't noticed while it was on the microfilm machine, with the headline: *New York Traveler Missing*.

"Hmm, this is interesting. Listen to this."

Lillian moved over next to her and looked over her shoulder while adjusting her glasses.

Laura read aloud, "County and State Health Department officials have called off the search for an unidentified male in his mid-30s from Saint Louis. Officials tracking the recent outbreak of smallpox in New York City, which has left twelve sick and two dead, are concerned the missing male may have been exposed to the infection while on a bus with a victim of the disease. The individual, described as Caucasian, tall, around 6 feet, 2 inches, with sandy-colored hair, mentioned to other bus riders that he intended to hike in the Adirondack mountains. The individual is presumed to be no longer in the local area."

"That's bizarre," Lillian said. "I wonder if they ever found the guy."

"Oh well," Laura said, "if it were anything other than smallpox, we might've actually hit on something. Do you mind if I use your phone? Bill wanted me to check in with him once I looked through the paper."

"No problem." Lillian put the phone on the counter.

"It'll just take a minute," Laura said, as she listened to numerous rings, but no answer. "I bet he's gone to bed. That rat - leaves me to do all the work, while he sleeps."

"Typical male," Lillian joked.

"You have a good night, Lillian – what's left of it." Laura patted Lillian on the arm. "Once again, I'm sorry I bothered you. I'll definitely be back to use the Internet."

"Okay, goodnight."

23

Bill awoke suddenly. It took a minute for him to realize where he was. Did he hear the phone ring? The kitchen light was still on, and the wall clock read three o'clock. The kink in his neck made him realize he'd fallen asleep at the kitchen table. There was no use fighting it. Without some rest now, there is no way he could tackle what he needed to do when the sun came up. As he headed toward the stairs to his bedroom, he wondered whether his father's death might've been a dream, so he peered into his father's room. Alfred's desk lamp dimly lit the area over the desk and surrounding floor. The pungent odor of blood mixed with the bleach that he'd sprayed earlier left no doubt of the grim reality. Fighting the urge to sleep, he decided he had better clean up the area instead. He pulled on some rubber gloves, grabbed a mop, a bucket, and some bleach solution out of the hallway closet.

As Bill mopped the floor, his mind drifted to childhood memories – learning to fish with his dad on Glacier Lake and hiking up Bald Peak together. He used to tag along with his dad at the office and saw patients with him as a teenager. Without that exposure at a young age, he would never have considered medicine as a career. His father had a magical way to put patients at ease and make them feel they had his full attention, regardless of their age or infirmity. He could inform someone of the most horrible diagnosis, but at the same time assure them of his undying support during their treatment and beyond.

Tears flowed freely down Bill's cheeks as he sponged the bathroom fixtures with bleach. He had missed the opportunity to resolve their differences. The least he could do now was to stop whatever scourge had taken him and stricken the town – he owed his father that much.

He put away the cleaning gear, washed his hands, and wiped his eyes with a towel. On the floor next to the desk, Bill spotted an ebony statue. He picked it up and noticed a fresh gash in place of a missing arm. A quick search under the desk revealed the arm. It matched the gash, so he resolved to find some glue whenever he could to repair it. As he reached to shut off the lamp, he noticed an old textbook with worn, yellowed pages left open on the desk. Without reading, he caught a glimpse of a disfigured child on the page before shutting off the lamp and leaving the room.

If he could just get another hour's sleep, he would be able to think more clearly. Just climbing the stairs took extraordinary effort. He wondered what horrific disease his father had been reading about – especially in an outdated textbook. He wasn't surprised that his father would be reading an old textbook – an outdated book for his father's outdated medical perspective. No surprise there, but it was too late to dwell on it. Without bothering to change his clothes, he fell onto his bed and drifted off to sleep - wondering what was taking Laura...

Bill fumbled in the dark and knocked the ringing phone off the nightstand. After searching the floor frantically, he finally picked up the receiver. "Hello?" he mumbled, half-awake.

"Dr. Denton. This is Lillian Johnson at the library. Your friend, Laura, just left. She piqued my curiosity, so I reviewed the microfilm again. I found another special bulletin the week before the ice storm. You were *right*! The town *was* put under quarantine because they feared a man travelling through the area might have smallpox."

"Uh huh," Bill managed to grunt, still semi-conscious and not completely understanding what she was talking about. "Sure, ice storm?" he mumbled.

Lillian explained further what she and Laura had found, and still half awake, Bill thanked her and hung up. He promptly fell back to sleep, but his subconscious mind repeated the word *smallpox*. Where had he seen that recently? Slowly, like a worm gnawing away at his brain, the picture of the child in his father's textbook came into focus. Suddenly, something in Bill's mind clicked. He opened his eyes. There was something all too familiar about that picture. He sat up.

"Laura?" he called out. Feeling a burst of adrenaline, he jumped off the bed and ran to Laura's room. It was empty. He bolted down the stairs and into the study, where he flicked on the desk light. Staring up at him from the open textbook was a child about the age of Jeremy Whitman. Large pustules covered his face and some coalesced into larger boils. The child's mouth was open in an anguished cry of pain. There was no doubt about it. His skin looked exactly like Jeremy's and Felicia's.

"Oh my God! Could it be?"

He read the chapter title, *Smallpox*. His eyes raced down the page, picking out key words as his adrenaline pumped. *After an average incubation period of 12-14 days, onset is sudden, with fever, headache, severe backache...a rash appears...there are several stages of the rash, from macules to papules, vesicles, and pustules*. His eyes froze on the next sentence: *there are more lesions on the face and the extremities than on the trunk*. He thought back to his discussions with Norm Phinney. He'd even said those exact words to Norm when he described the lesions on Jeremy Whitman and the frozen body. Bill's legs felt wobbly, as he collapsed onto the desk chair, but he forced himself to read on. *Approximately 3% of cases experienced a severe disease with a high fever and excessive bleeding...these cases, known as hemorrhagic smallpox or blackpox, were rapidly fatal*. His mind filled with visions of Jeremy Whitman bleeding on the night he coded. *The usual death rate was 15-40% in the unvaccinated, but symptoms could be much less severe or even non-existent in those previously vaccinated...often mistaken for varicella (chickenpox)*. He re-read the last line aloud, "Often mistaken for varicella." The words echoed in his head.

"SHIT!" he cried out. It couldn't be true. He banged the desk several times. "Oh my God," he repeated over and over. "How could I have been so blind?"

Laura rushed into the room. "Bill – what on earth is going on? I could hear your voice when I was pulling up outside."

"It's *smallpox*! Goddamn it! It's *smallpox*!"

"I know, the missing guy...the newspaper -"

"Not the newspaper – that's the disease!"

"What? You mean…wait, are you serious?"

"Do I look like I'm joking? I just got a call from Lillian. What did you guys find?"

"Nettie was right. The town closed down because of an ice storm. That's all. There was a small article about a guy who might have smallpox."

"There's more to it." Bill told her what he thought Lillian said on the phone. "You see? The town *was* put under quarantine. It must have been just before the ice storm. Look." He pointed to the textbook. "Read it. My dad left this page open. He must have suspected smallpox."

Bill paced the floor while Laura read.

"Oh my God!" Laura said. "This is horrible."

"You're telling me." Bill picked up the textbook - its pages smelled musty. "I thought it was quaint that my Dad would be reading an outdated textbook. But now I realize there is very little, if *anything* on smallpox in newer textbooks. That's probably why I didn't find anything about it in *my* books. After all, why do docs need to know about a disease that's vanished?"

Bill pulled the slip of paper out of his pocket that he'd written on just a couple of nights ago and re-read it:

Differential Diagnosis, Vesicular Rash

Smallpox was the third disease he'd written, and he'd drawn a line through it:

1) Chickenpox=varicella - may be deadly in

neonates and adults

2) Herpes simplex - generally localized, may be deadly in immunocompromised

~~*3) Smallpox - eradicated, 1980.*~~

3) Vesicular rickettsiosis - generally mild, transmitted by mites; no reported deaths

4) Drug reactions - what about vaccines?

5) Insect bites - could the children have had insect exposure?

"Damn!" Tears welled up in his eyes. Tears of anger, frustration, fear. "Look -" he showed the paper to Laura - "I even had it in my differential diagnosis. But since it was eradicated, I didn't even consider it. Damn! Damn!"

"Don't punish yourself," Laura said, grabbing his hands. "No one's seen it here for over 50 years. Who else would've recognized a case now or even thought to test for it? Your dad probably recognized it because of his experience in Africa before it was eradicated."

"That's right," Bill said, and he slapped the top of the desk. "Norm told me the lab had grown out a virus from the frozen body, but they couldn't identify it. That must be why. They probably don't even know how to test for it anymore."

"Exactly," Laura said. "The key is that you've recognized it *now*. Maybe we can do something to stop it."

"You're right. But before we sound the alarm, let's test our hypothesis. Does it really make sense with what's happened? The construction chief, Jed Thorton, had the highest possible exposure to the frozen body. He should've gotten sick, but he didn't. Thorton was the outlier. He's older than the others, so he must have been vaccinated. In fact, he used to be in the military, so I *know* he was vaccinated, probably more recently than even the rest of the population. The military continued vaccinating even after the civilians stopped."

"That's probably why the construction workers' kids got it, but fewer of the parents did. None of the kids would have been vaccinated."

"Makes sense to me," Bill said. "The parents probably received the vaccine as kids. Scott Gurnsey was different. He was too young. Mrs. Whitman didn't get sick either. Her parents were missionaries in Africa, where the disease continued for a while after it was eliminated in the United States, so no doubt she would've been vaccinated, probably multiple times."

"Definitely," said Laura.

"You know, now that I think about it," Bill said, "Jed Thorton told me that he'd been a bit under the weather and had some pimples. Maybe he just had a mild case. This is all starting to make sense. What about Norm Phinney? He cut himself. Even though he got sick from the cut, he never came down with smallpox. Why didn't *he* get it?"

"Beats me," said Laura. "Norm's probably too young to have been vaccinated before, and he probably wasn't in the military, like you."

"True, except he used to do research on viruses. Maybe he *was* vaccinated recently for his lab work. Let me see that book again."

Bill read that smallpox could be transmitted by several different means: through the air by small or large droplets, by direct contact with ill persons, and by fomites: inanimate objects, such as utensils, children's blocks, bed linen, and…contaminated clothes.

"I'll be damned! There it is," Bill said, tapping the page.

Laura read where he pointed and whistled.

"You were closer than you thought, after all," she said. "If those construction workers transmitted the infection to their kids by their contaminated clothes, that explains why they came down with it at the same time."

Bill stood silently, considering their options.

"Oh my God. Smallpox is such a horrible disease," Laura said. "It caused more deaths than any other disease in history, including things like the black death, typhoid, and cholera.

Bill saw images of hospital wards overflowing with rows-upon-rows of children's faces covered with pocks. Anguished cries of pain echoed through his mind.

"How do you know so much about smallpox?"

"I'm a history buff, remember? Smallpox is one of the more fascinating scourges, because it has so much historical importance. The vaccine against smallpox was the first vaccine ever discovered. Smallpox destroyed societies without immunity, like the Incas and Aztecs. It doesn't discriminate between the rich and poor. When half your population dies out quickly, there's a power vacuum, which leads to civil unrest and even war."

"So, this outbreak has enormous implications not only for this town, but for the whole world. This is an international emergency. Most of the world's population has no immunity, because we stopped vaccinating almost two decades ago after it was eradicated."

"We've got a virgin population, ready to be mown down."

"We're not going to let that happen. We've got to stop it," Bill said, as he darted back to the kitchen. Laura followed. "Let's start by spreading the word - the higher up the better. I'm calling the Centers for Disease Control. Someone should be there even at this hour."

After an endless series of phone pick lists, Bill thought he'd finally reached someone's private phone line. He gave Laura the "thumbs up" sign as the phone rang. Unfortunately, it turned out to be a voice mail machine. After the recording beep, he said, "This is Dr. Denton, from Elizabethtown, New York. I'm calling to report an outbreak of smallpox. That's right, *smallpox*. This is not a prank call. This is an emergency. Please call me back as soon as you receive this message." He left his home, office, and cell phone numbers.

Bill tried the number several more times, each time punching in different numbers when prompted. He still couldn't reach anyone, so he finally gave up.

"It's clear that's getting nowhere. Let's go to plan B."

"What's plan B?" Laura asked.

"I don't have a clue. Got any suggestions?"

"When we *do* finally reach someone, won't they be skeptical? I mean, why would they believe us?"

"Yeah, hmm – sort of like saying you've raised Lazarus from the dead."

"It would be a lot easier to convince someone if we had laboratory proof. What about Norm? Would he have anything we could use?"

"It doesn't hurt to find out."

Norm's phone rang at least eight times before he answered.

"Norm, this is Bill."

"Who?" Norm mumbled, sounding half-asleep.

"Bill...Bill Denton."

"Oh…sorry. I'm not used to getting calls at this hour. What time is it anyway?"

Bill looked at his watch. "Three-thirty."

"Damn! What the hell?"

Bill explained his discovery.

"Are you shitting me?"

"No, but trust me. Remember the lab grew something from that frozen body, but couldn't identify it? How could they? They probably don't even have the right lab tests to identify it anymore. Most lab technicians probably weren't even born when we were testing for it."

"You've got a point there," Norm said. "So, what do you want me to do?"

"You said the viral sample was forwarded from Saranac Lake to the state reference lab. Where is that?"

"Albany."

"Call them. Find out what they know, and whether

they referred it somewhere else. What's the fastest way that a lab could diagnose smallpox?"

"Probably with an electron microscope. But those are only at large research centers. PCR's another way, but most small labs wouldn't have the right primers or reagents to do PCR, either. The bottom line is if the Albany lab can't make a diagnosis, they'll have to send it to the CDC in Atlanta."

"Great. Call them and find out."

"Hold on, man. It's 3:30 in the morning. I have no idea how to contact the lab at this hour. It's going to have to wait until later this morning."

"It can't, pal. Every minute counts. I don't care what you have to do, but you find the director of the lab at home. Find out wherever this specimen went and make sure it gets tested in Albany or sent to the CDC ASAP. Call me when you reach someone."

"Ok, but I have no idea how to do this."

"You're a big boy, Norm. You'll figure it out." Bill hung up and then updated Laura on the conversation.

"We've got to get some data to convince the CDC about what's going on, but it could take a day or two before we get that lab result back. If smallpox is as infectious as I think, there's no time to lose. Anyone who works on that specimen could get infected."

"Consider this," Laura said, "the empires I mentioned before were decimated long before air travel. Imagine how much worse things will be now. This thing could already be incubating halfway around the globe. What's our next move?"

"We don't have time to wait until Norm reaches the lab in Albany or gets that specimen to the CDC. He said only a few types of labs could make the diagnosis. There's got to be another way around this." He drummed his fingers on the kitchen table. "Wait!" He banged the table, startling Laura. "I've got it! Norm left out one key type of laboratory."

Laura lifted up her hands as if to say "What?"

"A military lab?"

"They have the capabilities?"

"Definitely. You remember my friend Martinez?" Laura nodded. "He works at USAMRIID – the U.S. Army Medical Research Institute of Infectious Diseases. They have the pre-eminent maximum containment labs in the country. They develop vaccines against the world's most horrific infectious diseases. You remember that book, *Inside the Hot Zone*?"

"Yeah – the one about anthrax, Ebola, and biological warfare?"

"Exactly. USAMRIID is the Army's biological warfare defense laboratory. They've hunted down all sorts of outbreaks, from Hantavirus Pulmonary Syndrome in the southwest US, to Rift Valley fever in Egypt. They're like the country's *Biohazard 9-1-1* – an emergency hotline when you've been hit with some horrible infectious disease. Martinez is well connected across the globe, and he has friends at the CDC. Hell, half the people in the Special Pathogens Branch at the CDC used to work at USAMRIID. If I can convince Martinez this is smallpox, he'll know what to do. I'll get him on the phone STAT."

24

Bill's call pulled Martinez out of a deep slumber. Once Martinez was fully awake, Bill explained the situation and described the victims.

"You know, Bill," Martinez said, "I've never lent much credence to those doomsayers who have worried that smallpox could re-emerge from a victim unearthed from the permafrost, but your ice cave story sounds compelling. The illness *does* sound consistent with smallpox."

"So, what can you do?"

"Don't take this the wrong way, buddy," Martinez said. "I trust your clinical instincts, but before we pull the trigger, we need some proof. Declaring a smallpox outbreak, if it ain't that, could send global shockwaves and we'd look like fools. Before I call in a *Biohazard 9-1-1*, our nickname for a global outbreak emergency, I need to get eyes on those patients who are here in Washington, DC. I live about 15 minutes from downtown and I just happen to have an infectious disease colleague who works at that hospital. I'll give him some warning, but I don't think he'll mind if I drop in on those patients with him. What are their names again?"

"The Whitmans – Michelle and Otis."

"Right. If they look even remotely like they've got smallpox, then we're all up a creek, and I'd alert my USAMRIID commander, then the CDC, the WHO, and any other God damned place in the world I can think of. Ok?"

"Sounds good."

"Give me about an hour," Martinez said. "I'll call you as soon as I see them."

"Great. Thanks, buddy."

Bill hung up the phone and updated Laura. "Now we're getting somewhere," he said. "Let's go wake up the mayor. It's time for him to earn his pay."

Once on the road, Bill used his cell phone to call

Henry O'Donnell and alerted him of their impending arrival. The mayor reluctantly agreed to meet with them.

By now the moon had slid behind a mountain, leaving the night pitch black, except for the road and the passing evergreens moving in and out of the beam of the headlights. Bill didn't feel talkative as he contemplated meeting with the mayor.

"It's strange," Laura said, breaking the silence. "It's so peaceful at this time of night, yet we might be on the verge of a major catastrophe."

"The deathly calm before the storm," Bill said. "I think we've already passed beyond the verge."

"Do you think that frozen body could be the same guy who disappeared after that New York City epidemic?"

"I don't know, but it would certainly tie everything together nicely. The whole thing's completely bizarre."

"Half the town could be incubating this disease right now," Laura said. "In the 1970s, a German electrician who visited Pakistan was admitted to a hospital in Germany, with a diagnosis of typhoid fever."

"Oh, yeah. I think I remember reading about that case when I was in the Army. It's a famous case study. I seem to recall when they eventually realized it was smallpox instead, they moved him to a specialized smallpox hospital and immediately vaccinated everyone at the first hospital – patients and staff alike, but there were more cases, right?

"Yes," said Laura. "Another 18 people still became sick."

"That's it. Isn't that the one that spread by the air?"

"Yes. They mapped out where all the cases occurred – some were two floors above where the original patient stayed! They couldn't figure it out…until they released smoke in his room and followed where it went. The air currents carried it all through that wing of the hospital."

"That's the story. I remember it now. Damn!" Bill hit the steering wheel. "So, this stuff can infect someone downwind or through a ventilation system. Oh man. We are *screwed*!"

They were both quiet again for a few minutes until Laura broke the silence.

"I'm really scared."

Bill reached over and patted her hand. "I know. So am I, but we have to focus. We can't let it get to us. We have to believe we'll get through this."

"You don't understand. I…I was never vaccinated."

Bill caught his breath. *Oh, God*, he thought. He hadn't even considered that Laura might get sick. He could barely steer the car as his hands began to tremble.

"They stopped vaccinating before I was born. I was exposed to your dad and probably also from your clothes. I'm a ticking time bomb."

"No, you're not." Bill hoped what he said was true. "Look. Martinez is on the case. Once he confirms that this is smallpox, they'll throw all sorts of vaccine our way. If you haven't gotten sick yet, there must be a reason. You'll get vaccinated in time to prevent the disease. Don't let it get the better of you. Besides," he squeezed her hand, "I'm really going to need your help."

Laura managed a weak smile, barely visible in the glow of the dashboard. "How about you – you were vaccinated, right?"

"Yes," Bill answered. "I didn't have a choice. When I was in the military it was mandatory, and I've got a scar to prove it. Maybe that's why I haven't gotten sick yet."

"During the eradication campaign," Laura said, "they gave people booster vaccines every three years in the countries where there was a lot of transmission. The immunity can last up to five to ten years, or maybe even longer if someone gets vaccinated several times."

As they approached Elizabethtown, they drove past several quiet, dark, lonely houses. Just on the outskirts, Bill took a left turn onto a dirt road that coursed along the side of

Cobble Hill. The mayor's log cabin was the first driveway on the right. As Bill pulled in, the porch lights turned on. At the same time, Bill's cell phone went off. It was Norm.

"Bill, I reached the lab manager at the state public health lab in Albany. The specimen was still there, but they couldn't identify the organism. I told the manager he had to ship it shipped to the CDC as soon as possible. He said he'd do what he could, but the earliest he could get a courier was later today."

"All right, Norm." Bill updated him on his conversation with Martinez. "Laura and I just arrived at the mayor's house. Keep pushing it, and we'll meet you at the hospital when we're done here."

Bill and Laura got out of the car and were swarmed by black flies and moths around the porch lights. The mayor stepped out onto the porch wearing a bathrobe, which partially covered his light blue pajama top and bottom, but it couldn't hide his large gut.

"This better be good, Doc."

"I wouldn't wake you up for nothing," Bill said, as he stepped onto the porch.

The mayor ushered them into a spacious living room lit by a deer antler chandelier. Large beams crisscrossed the vaulted ceiling, and throw rugs were scattered about the oak hard wood floor.

"Keep your voices low," Henry said. "I don't want to disturb my wife – she has a bad headache."

Bill and Laura sat on an oversized brown leather sofa, while the mayor took a wooden rocker opposite them.

"Okay, Doc," Henry said. "What's so God-damned important?"

Even though Bill knew he was doing the right thing, Henry was still incredibly intimidating. The mantra in the military is: *bottom line up front*. He suspected that would be the best approach with Henry - give him the key information and then let him chew on it.

"The illness that you came to see me about. I believe it's smallpox. If I'm right, then this is an international emergency."

"Smallpox?" Henry repeated the word a couple times to himself, as if trying to jog his memory. "What the hell is that?"

"It was a devastating worldwide disease that can cause a horrific rash and kills about thirty percent of its victims."

"Wait, is that the vaccine that leaves a scar?"

"Yes," said Bill. "You probably received it as a kid."

"Wait a minute," Henry said. "Wasn't that wiped out or somethin'?"

"Yes," said Laura.

"In 1980," said Bill.

"This is crazy. How does something like that come back?"

Bill explained his theory about the frozen corpse.

"You *think* it's smallpox, but you're not sure?"

"That's right."

"When will you know?"

"Hopefully very soon – within the next couple of hours." Bill told him about Martinez.

"This is horse shit!" Henry hoisted his heavy from his chair and paced back and forth, muttering to himself and slamming his fist into his hand repeatedly. "You woke me up for this? Fanciful stories about a disease that was wiped out almost two decades ago? This sounds like something out of a dime-store novel. I've got too much going on for this kind of crap."

Laura's expression betrayed her shock and fear. Bill felt his anger building.

"I'm trying to put this town on the map again, and everywhere I turn, I get stymied. This is all I *God damn* need right now." The mayor pointed a finger at Bill. "Get out of here! Don't bother me again unless you've got some proof or

I'm gonna kick your ass out of town – yours and your girlfriend's."

Bill could no longer contain himself. He jumped up and grabbed Henry's arm. "Damn you!" he yelled directly in his face. "This could be the worst health crisis in a century, and all you care about is your fucking resort? Go to hell! If you won't help us, then we'll go it alone. Let's get out of here." Bill grabbed Laura's hand and they practically ran out the door.

As they were jumping off the porch, Henry yelled after them. "Denton, get back here! No one walks out on me like that."

Bill stopped and turned slowly back toward Henry, who stood in the doorway with a shotgun trained on him. "Oh, Henry, that's *real* good. That'll solve everything." He waved Laura toward the car. Laura ran over and jumped into the car. "You think that gun scares me? You think no one's threatened me before in some of the shitholes where I've deployed? You need me. You can't stop this thing without me, so just put the gun down and I'll forget this ever happened." Henry just stood there, with his mouth agape. "I'll get you proof, Henry. Then I'll call the undertaker to bury your sorry ass along with all the other victims caused by your stalling."

Bill turned and slowly stepped off the porch, cringing in anticipation of feeling a blast in his back. If he moved slowly enough, maybe Henry wouldn't pull the trigger. Gravel on the driveway crunched under his feet with each step. Henry's heavy breathing sounded as if it was just behind his right ear. Bill reached the car and opened the door slowly. He got in and started the engine. The tires spun as he jammed his foot down on the accelerator. In his rearview mirror, he caught a glimpse of Henry at the edge of his driveway shaking his fist at him.

"I really thought he might use that thing," Laura said.

"Me, too."

Bill noticed that he had missed a call from Martinez.

He tried to call him back, but his hands were shaking too much. He handed the phone to Laura, "Can you punch in the numbers for me?" Too angry and upset to talk and drive at the same time, he pulled over to the side of the dirt road. When Martinez answered, Laura put the phone on speaker.

"Bill," Martinez said, "I've seen the Whitmans. They sure as hell look like they've got a classic case of smallpox, although I might have missed the diagnosis without being primed. They even have this peculiar stench that I've read about from all the decaying flesh. I've already spoken with Jim Hayworth, the CDC director and my boss, Colonel Etson, the USAMRIID commander. Some other things can be mistaken for smallpox, especially hemorrhagic smallpox, so they don't want to sound the alarm until they can confirm the diagnosis with a lab sample, but the CDC's already dusting off their plans to mobilize vaccine, if necessary. There are two confirmation laboratories for handling bioterrorism specimens: the CDC and USAMRIID. Since USAMRIID's just outside Washington, DC, I plan to rush the samples there as we speak. USAMRIID's already mobilizing its AIT to collect them."

"The AIT?" Bill asked.

"The Aeromedical Isolation Team - an 8-person team with a doc and a nurse who are well trained in dealing with the most horrific viruses on the planet. They've been mobilized in the past to help out with Ebola outbreaks, and they have a special mobile isolation unit that can transport a patient or a sample under maximum Bio-Safety Level 4 containment to minimize the chances that this virus can get out while in transit. They're going to fly down in a Blackhawk helicopter and bring the samples back to USAMRIID."

"Is all that necessary?" Bill asked. "I mean, it's only about a 45-minute drive from USAMRIID down to DC. Can't they just drive down and pick them up?"

"Sure, but just imagine the political fallout if someone highjacked the car or if the virus got out. How many governors would let them drive through their state with a package like that?"

"You've got a point there," Bill said. "By the way, did the docs taking care of the Whitmans suspect smallpox?"

"No, but believe it or not, a third-year medical student mentioned it in her differential diagnosis at a staff conference a couple days ago and the staff blew her off. I thought my buddy there was going to shit in his pants when I told him about it."

"Damn, Martinez, I guess that makes me feel a little better that I'm not the only one who missed the diagnosis."

"No, pal. Don't sweat it. If you hadn't alerted us, it might have taken another week to get anyone thinking about that, and then another day or two to convince anyone it was real. You've bought us valuable time."

"What kind of isolation did they have the Whitmans under?" Bill asked.

"That's the bad news. Only enteric precautions – you know, washing hands frequently and minimizing contact with human waste on top of the usual precautions against blood contact. They thought they were dealing with typhoid fever. Anyone who's set foot in that wing of the building since yesterday could've been exposed, especially because Michelle Whitman was coughing a lot. All those people are going to need to be vaccinated – we're talking at *least* a few hundred people. The hospital CEO was pissed when I told him."

"I can imagine. Thanks for the update. Let me know what they find at USAMRIID, and when we should expect some vaccine. I'll have a lot of anxious people here once the word gets out."

"Ten-four."

Bill shut off the phone and looked at Laura. "This is a disaster. It's eerily similar to that case study you mentioned of the German electrician with smallpox, who was *also* mistaken for having typhoid fever. We need to start planning a massive campaign to vaccinate the town, with or without Henry."

As he started to pull back onto the road, Bill's cell phone went off again. It was the Emergency Room.

"Dr. Denton," the voice on the other line said, "two patients just came in with high fevers and may need to be admitted. Can you see them?"

Bill felt a knot in his stomach. After a slight hesitation, he said, "I'll be right there." Then he shut off the phone.

Laura grabbed his arm. "What's going on?"

"This is just the beginning. I'm afraid it's the second wave."

25

Martinez stepped into the locker room for Animal Assessment Room 5, a Biosafety Level 4 laboratory inside USAMRIID, where he stripped out of his street clothes and donned a pair of scrub tops and bottoms along with socks. He walked through a dry shower area into the "gray" area of the laboratory, a transition zone between the safe hallway outside the lab and the "hot" side of the lab where he worked on deadly pathogens. Here he taped his socks to his scrubs and then taped a pair of surgical gloves to his long sleeve scrub top. Next, he partially inflated his blue "space suit" and inspected it for leaky holes and cracks. Once everything looked good, he placed earplugs into his ears. Next, like putting on a fireman's gear, he first stepped into the suit's foot compartment at the base of the suit, then pulled it up around his waist, followed by sliding his left arm into the sleeve. Then he ducked his head in and slid his right arm into the other sleeve with a single motion. Once fully inside the suit, he pulled the large zipper down across his chest, sealing himself inside. He hooked up the air pressure valve to the side of his suit and felt a rush of cool air over the top of his head. At this point, he couldn't hear much except the hiss of the air and his own breathing, but he was now ready to head into the hot side of the lab.

He pushed the green button on the wall next to the large stainless steel shower door and waited for the rubber gaskets around the door to deflate and the light next to the button to turn from red to green, indicating it was safe to enter. He pulled the large door open and stepped into the decontamination shower. Because he was headed *into* the lab, he didn't need to undergo decontamination, but he would do so when it came time to exit the lab. He hooked up to the air hose in the shower while waiting for the green light to signal it was okay to open the door on the opposite side of the shower. As he opened the door into the lab, he felt the hushed stillness inside. He unplugged the shower air hose, and was enveloped in a moment of silence, until he reattached to a new air hose in the hallway and once again felt a rush of air. He was now on the "hot" side of the lab, where he conducted work with deadly viruses. He closed the stainless-steel shower door behind him and pushed a button to start a decontamination cycle inside the shower.

He pulled on a pair of fireman's green rubber boots, unhooked the air hose and shuffled down the central lab corridor until he reached the lab room that housed an electron microscope. He stepped into the lab and hooked up again to a new air hose. Martinez had obtained a specimen from one of the pustules on Michelle Whitman's chest. His technician, Tom, was already in the lab working with the specimen.

He didn't want to surprise Tom while he was working, so he tapped Tom on the shoulder in case he hadn't noticed Martinez enter. Tom gave him a wave. Picking up a handheld, dry erase board, Tom wrote, "Almost ready." Martinez responded with a thumbs up.

Martinez rolled over a stool, so he could sit behind Tom and view the glowing green screen of the electron microscope as he worked. Once everything was set, Tom loaded Michelle's specimen into the chamber where the electron beam of the microscope would penetrate it. Then he fiddled with several dials until an image on the screen below came into focus.

It didn't take long for Martinez to recognize the classic shapes of an orthopoxvirus, like the smallpox virus. The specimen was teaming with them: like rectangles or pineapples, with rounded, corrugated edges, which some have also described as brick-like structures. They were so numerous and the structures so obvious, Martinez thought a 5-year-old could recognize them. There were many different orthopoxviruses that could look like this under an electron microscope in addition to smallpox: monkeypox, Orf, cowpox, and vaccinia. But no other orthopoxvirus could cause the severity of disease and rapid demise of so many people and be linked to a body in the permafrost. This *had* to be smallpox. Over the course of his career, Martinez dealt with contagion on three continents, but never something like this. He said a quiet prayer to himself and made the cross symbol across his chest.

Tom gazed at Martinez, with a wide-eyed look of horror. Martinez acknowledged it and gave Tom a reassuring tap on the shoulder. Martinez knew what he had to do. It was time to sound the alarm. He beat a hasty retreat back through the lab. As he stood in the decon shower during its seven-minute cycle feeling the cool decontaminating solution spraying all around him, followed by a warm water rinse, he rehearsed his plan of attack. First, he would alert his commanding general, who could carry the ball up the military chain of command to the Chairman of the Joint Chiefs of Staff. Then he would phone his friend, the CDC director, and the two of them could go straight to the Chief of Staff at the White House. There was no time to waste. Once dressed, he rushed down the hall to the USAMRIID headquarters to call in a Biohazard 9-1-1.

26

The Emergency Room waiting area was abuzz with people. By the time Bill arrived, the contract ER doc on call, Joel Brown, had at least two more patients lined up to see him. He guided Bill and Laura into the conference room at the back of the ER.

"Bill," Brown said, "ever since Jeremy Whitman died, the nurses are on edge. One of the guys waiting to see you works here in the lab. The staff suspects he accidentally infected himself while handling specimens from Jeremy. They're spreading rumors that this might be Ebola or something."

"I understand," Bill said. "Please gather everyone together, and I'll explain what's going on."

"Okay." Brown left.

"Bill," Laura said, "while you're seeing the patients, I'll put together a vaccination strategy."

"Great."

The hospital staff began to arrive. Once everyone was seated, Bill explained his concern about smallpox and his discussions with Washington, DC. He read the fear in their eyes.

"In the meantime, while we're waiting for confirmation, we need to do a couple things. Any patient who walks in the door gets a surgical mask; I don't care whether or not they look sick. If we have enough N-95 masks, anyone seeing a patient needs to wear one. Smallpox is an extremely severe and deadly infection." The staff had a variety of expressions to this – some quizzical, others nonchalant. "This disease, if it *is* smallpox, spreads mainly by close contact with respiratory secretions. If we can protect our respiratory tracts and our mucus membranes, then we can decrease our risk of infection. How many here have been vaccinated against smallpox?"

The staff was relatively young. Only about a third of them raised their hand.

"Until we get vaccine," Bill said, "I want only those who've previously been vaccinated to care for anyone with a fever or a rash."

One of the older nurses raised her hand. "How do we know if the vaccine we had will do any good?"

Bill sensed the potential for the situation to spin out of control. "I have to be honest with you," he said, "the vaccine may protect you for ten years, perhaps even longer. I can't say for sure how long. We have to assume that whatever immunity some of us had in the past has waned. It may no longer completely prevent disease, but it might make the disease less severe and hopefully prevent death. That's why we must take extra precautions with masks, and wear gowns and gloves when seeing any patients."

"I don't want to take care of these patients." the nurse said. "I've got kids, and I can't afford to get sick."

"Yeah," another staff member piped in, "I'm getting out of here." The situation in the room quickly turned into chaos as everyone spoke at once.

"Hold on everyone!" Bill shouted as he raised his hands and stood up on a chair. "Let me have your attention." The room quieted down. "Remember. We're *all* medical providers. *We* are the ones who know how disease spreads, and how to limit that spread. You -" Bill pointed directly at some of the staff closest to him - "you can have a great influence on how the rest of the town reacts to this. And without you, there will be no one to care for you or your family members if *you or they* get sick. Do you want that to happen? If others in town see you panicking, they're going to freak. If this town turns into chaos, there's no way we can vaccinate anyone or respond effectively to whatever will occur."

The staff appeared to be temporarily satisfied, although they continued to whisper and some of their faces revealed fear.

Bill said, "Another thing we need to do is control access into the hospital. Otherwise, people could wander in and expose themselves or staff elsewhere in the building. Judy-" Bill singled out the tall, blond chief nurse in the back of the room - "contact the sheriff. We'll need one of his deputies assigned to stand guard at the hospital for the time being. We'll also have to lock some of the side entrances." Judy nodded. "Does anyone have any questions?"

"What can we do with these patients?" the ER clerk asked.

"There is no treatment," Bill answered, "so the best thing we can do is give them information and try to reassure them. We may not be able to cure them, but we can still show them we care. If one person in a family is ill, chances are the rest of their family's already been exposed. For those who are not severely ill, by sending them home in the care of their family, we can limit the potential for spread to others in the community. Our strategy will be to vaccinate the remaining healthy family members as soon as possible, to try and prevent them from getting infected."

"But don't you need the vaccine before you get exposed? Isn't it too late afterward?" the clerk asked again.

"That's a very good question," Bill answered. "Yes, because the time it takes to become ill after being exposed, the incubation period, is longer than the time it takes to get protection from the vaccine. That means if we can get you vaccinated soon, you can be protected even after you've been exposed. Miss Chen, would you care to elaborate regarding the global smallpox eradication effort?" Bill turned toward Laura.

"Yes Dr. Denton," Laura responded. "During the smallpox eradication effort, they used a strategy called *surveillance and containment*. Once they identified someone with smallpox, they vaccinated everyone within a certain radius of that infected person – so-called *ring vaccination*.

The key factor, though, was speed. The quicker people got vaccinated, the better their chance of disrupting the infection."

"Thanks, Laura," Bill said. "The bottom line is: we've already had two terminal patients in this hospital. Chances are that many of you have already been exposed."

There were a couple of gasps from the staff. Bill held up his right hand to suppress the whispering.

"Yes. It's shocking, but I must be frank with you. We could *all* be incubating this disease right now - me included. The important thing is that the vaccine can help us as soon as we get it, but we need to maintain order. We have an obligation as health care professionals to take care of sick people. The best way to help your loved ones and your patients is to remain calm and do what we've been trained to do. We *can* prevent further infection by simple measures such as masks and gloves. So, let's get out there and take care of these people."

The staff began to filter out of the room.

Bill turned to Laura. "Thanks for that input. I think it helped to allay their fears a little. Time will tell."

Bill's phone rang. It was Martinez. As Bill grabbed his phone, he told Dr. Brown he'd be out momentarily to help with the patients.

"What's up Martinez?" Bill asked.

"USAMRIID's determined with electron microscopy that this *is* an orthopoxvirus. I've seen it with my own eyes! That means it's either smallpox or one of its close cousins, like monkeypox. They'll have some confirmatory PCR results in a couple hours."

"Great. So, what now?"

"I've been on calls with the White House, the FBI, USAMRIID, the CDC, Homeland Security, and you name it. It's a dumpster fire. They're working out a strategy how best to use the vaccine. Since it's a live virus vaccine, if someone has AIDS, or leukemia, or takes steroids, or is otherwise immune suppressed, they can have a terrible reaction - even die - from the vaccine alone."

"I know," Bill said. "In other words, we have to be judicious about how we use it."

"Exactly." Martinez said. "They're working out how best to target the people who need it the most. They've had drills before for something like this, but the real situation is always more complicated. The problem is that the number of potentially infected people is expanding exponentially. Michelle Whitman, with her cough, was probably a very efficient vector and exposed a whole plane-full of people, a hotel-full of people, and potentially thousands of people visiting the Smithsonian and the Capitol. Those people have probably dispersed all across the country or even the world by now and could expose more people."

"What are you trying to tell me?"

"It's scary, Bill. This is going to be hard to get a handle on. You think tracking the slow roll of HIV was tough. That was child's play compared to this, due to the rapid spread. It's going to take a good chunk of the CDC and the state and county health departments all across this country to rein this thing in. The FBI's worried about bioterrorism. There's talk that the North Koreans or al Qaeda may have unleashed this."

"Wait a second," said Bill, "I told you where this all started. What do you mean bioterrorism?"

"Exactly what I said. I've told them your story, but no one buys it. Smallpox is on the CDC's category A threat list. It's the perfect bioweapon, so they're assuming this was released by a terrorist until proven otherwise."

"That's ridiculous!"

"Hey, I hear you, pal," Martinez said, "but this is an international crisis. All the different factions that handle these kinds of things are jockeying for position. We're talking a major pissing contest. The CDC and FBI are already fighting over who's in charge."

"Okay, listen. I can't worry about that stuff. My job is to save this town. When do I get the vaccine?" Bill asked.

"I don't know. I've got a meeting in a few minutes. The CDC's going to outline their plan of action. I'll let you know more later. Watch for a press conference from the President shortly."

"Okay. Keep me in the loop. Get me that vaccine!" Bill hung up, and then he updated Laura.

"This thing's already out of control," Laura said.

"You're telling me," Bill said. "What have you come up with?"

"I think the high school gym's the best place to hold a vaccine party," Laura said. "It's large enough, centrally located, and we could control access. I've already coordinated everything with the principal."

"Great. Do you know how to give the vaccine?"

"They don't teach it in nursing school anymore, but I've read about it - seems pretty basic. You just dip a bifurcated needle into the vaccine liquid and then do 3 pokes with it on the upper arm. The needle's designed to extract just the right amount of vaccine between its two prongs."

"Great. You'll be the lead vaccinator. You can train the other nurses and me when the time comes. I'm off to see the patients now."

27

Bill pulled on an N-95 mask to protect himself from inhaling contagion. His first patient was a 20-year-old male who worked in the hospital laboratory and had a 102-degree fever with muscle and backaches. Bill didn't see any signs of a rash yet, but he suspected it would soon appear. The man remembered processing lab samples for Jeremy Whitman, and one of the glass tubes had shattered, splashing blood around the lab, giving him a potential exposure. Two other patients were classmates of Jeremy Whitman, both with fevers above 100 degrees the day before and now each had small bumps on their faces. The fourth patient was Jeremy's teacher, a 25-year-old woman who appeared the sickest of them all. She had a fever, severe backache, and had vomited several times. Small bumps, like pimples in the early stages, had multiplied on her face. She felt much better after Bill inserted an intravenous catheter and gave her some IV fluids, but he knew her relief would be temporary.

One-by-one, Bill sent the patients home with as much reassurance as he could, knowing he had nothing more to offer them in the hospital than what they could get at home. Without a specific treatment, their outcome was really between them and God. Before sending anyone home, he verified that all patients had someone who could care for them in their home, and he stressed the importance of getting family members vaccinated as soon as the vaccine became available. He also counseled family members on how to protect themselves from getting infected, even if there was a chance they were already infected. He also gave them masks and gloves to protect them. He made a list of the patients, with their phone numbers and addresses, so their family members could be followed up for vaccination.

As Bill finished up with the last patient, one of the nurses called everyone to the waiting room. The President appeared on the television for a press conference. His face was red, and he had dark rings under his eyes. He stuttered his words and shifted his stance continually.

"Hey, Bill," Dr. Brown said, "the President doesn't look so good."

"You wouldn't either if you had to save the world from smallpox."

Bill looked around the room. Everyone's attention was laser focused on the television.

"Mr. President," a reporter asked, "didn't the World Health Organization certify the world free of smallpox in 1980 and that the only known stores of smallpox virus are held at the CDC and in Russia? How could this happen?"

"Right now, I can share that two suspected cases have been admitted to a Washington, DC hospital," the President answered. "We are conferring with the experts at the CDC and USAMRIID at Fort Detrick on the best way to handle the situation. We are taking the appropriate measures. We have preliminary indications that this is smallpox, but we are waiting on confirmatory laboratory test results from USAMRIID."

Bill was amazed how fast all of this had happened. He admired how influential Martinez must have been to sound the alarm. It couldn't have been more than two or three hours since he'd first told Martinez about smallpox. Bill noticed on the stage with the President was the CDC Director and just behind her was Martinez.

"The CDC's investigation into potential spread has already begun," the President said. "I want to assure everyone that we have the situation under control."

"Mr. President," another reporter asked, "How many doses of smallpox vaccine do we have in the U.S. stockpile?"

"I've been assured that we have enough to vaccinate everyone in the United States, if the disease is confirmed as smallpox," the President answered.

Another reporter jumped in. "With all due respect,

Sir, during the last major epidemic of smallpox in New York City, in 1947, they burned through over 6 million doses to vaccinate just the population of the city. The numbers can add up fast, especially if you consider potential wastage of the vaccine."

The President's face turned redder. "We have enough, but we can also manufacture more doses if we need to. Please wait until I recognize you before you ask a question. Next question...Yes?" He pointed to another reporter.

"Sir, can you comment on the rumor that congressional members were exposed when one of the victims visited the Capitol this week?"

The President appeared caught off guard. Bill wondered if he hadn't been briefed about that yet. "I..." the President stammered, "I can't address that until our experts at the CDC and the Washington, D.C. Health Department assess the situation. I will ensure that the information gets disseminated as soon as possible. Once again, I want to assure the American people and our friends abroad that we are taking this seriously. Before I close, let me apprise you of the measures that have already been taken in the past several years for a potential act of bioterrorism such as this. Rapid surveillance systems and a laboratory network have been put in place across the country to identify unusual clusters of disease. We are taking all the necessary steps to contain this outbreak using those tools. As soon as the disease is confirmed, I will update you. Thank you, and God bless America." The President left the podium abruptly, followed by shouts with additional questions from the reporters.

The medical staff in the waiting room all began talking at once. Someone said, "You hear that? They don't have enough vaccine."

"I'm getting out of here," another said.

"I can't take this!" someone else yelled.

People started running in different directions. Bill shouted, "That's not what the President said," but it was no use. The staff grabbed whatever they could of their belongings and left. Bill tried to stop a couple as they ran for the door, but to no avail. Even the deputy sheriff guarding the entrance bolted. Bill stood alone at the ER entrance, watching the different employees jump into their cars, and hearing them gun their engines. A couple of them nearly crashed into each other in their mad dash out of the parking lot. Bill returned to the waiting room where Laura sat alone with a vacant stare and tears streaming down her cheeks. Bill walked over to the television and turned it off.

"So, what now?" Laura asked in between tearful gasps.

Bill held her hands and pulled her arms around him. They hugged for a long time, and then Bill grabbed a tissue off an end table. He dabbed Laura's tears. Her sobs diminished. "I guess it's just you and me," he said.

Dr. Brown walked in. "I left for a minute to check on some labs. Where the hell is everyone?"

"They've all checked out, and I doubt they're coming back."

"Crap. At this point, they've probably all been exposed, so running home isn't going to help. In fact, it's a great opportunity to spread it to more people."

"Yeah," Bill said. "Well, listen, at least we have the three of us."

"And one of the nurses is still hanging around on the wards," Brown said, "as well as one guy in the lab."

"Okay. That's better than nothing. Let's start by reassessing what *we* can do together. What arrangements did you make with the principal?" Bill asked Laura.

"We can use the gym any time. School's canceled until further notice. Unfortunately, the deputy principal has a headache and fever, too." Laura's tearful eyes couldn't mask her fear. "Bill, tell me honestly. Do you think they have enough *Dryvax*?"

"*Dryvax*?"

"Smallpox vaccine. That's a brand name."

"Oh." Bill had an odd feeling. The name seemed somehow familiar. "I don't know. We'll find out soon. The vaccine's the key to quelling the panic." Bill scratched his head. "Hmm, you mentioned *Dryvax*. I think I've heard or seen that word somewhere recently."

"That's not surprising," Brown said. "Maybe you were reading a textbook or something online?"

"I don't know. I don't think so. I haven't read about smallpox in a long time, and not recently until I read my dad's textbook. I doubt they'd mention a brand name for the vaccine in any of the older book chapters. No. I know I've seen it somewhere else recently. But where?"

Bill put his face in his hands, trying to concentrate. He could almost visualize a vial with the words on it. But where had he seen it?

Laura sat down next to him and put her arm on his shoulder. "Maybe somewhere here in the hospital? Norm Phinney's office?"

"Office!" Bill said and jumped up off the couch. "That's it! My dad's office."

"At home?"

"No – the clinic," Bill said. "Damn! I remember seeing it now - in the freezer. Let's go."

Bill started to move but then stopped. "Wait. Joel, I don't want to leave you abandoned here by yourself. Can you hold the fort down here for a while? I still have a couple of patients. They're stable, though."

"Relax, Bill, I'm an ER doc. I'm used to multi-tasking in a crisis. I can handle things here, and I'll have the nurse and lab tech to help me. You do what you need to do."

"Okay," Bill said. "You've got my cell phone and pager numbers. If you get overwhelmed, I'll come back."

"No problemo," Brown said.

Bill and Laura left and drove to the clinic as fast as possible. The center of town was a mob scene. People were gunning their way through the central intersection without stopping. Bill narrowly avoided getting side swiped during the short drive.

"A couple weeks ago," Bill said, "I was looking in the freezer for some viral media to culture a patient's skin lesion. I saw a vial of *Dryvax* in the freezer. It was right in front of my eyes. I had no idea what it was then. I meant to ask Rosemary about it, but I forgot."

"That's great! Maybe that's how we can stop this thing," Laura said. "How many vials?"

"I think only one, but if my dad saved one, maybe he saved more. How many doses are there in one vial?"

"I think it's supposed to be somewhere between 60 to 100 doses. You might be able to stretch it if you're careful and use a bifurcated needle."

"Wow! That could be enough for about a fifth of the town. If we targeted those at highest risk of infection, it might be enough to establish some herd immunity and interrupt transmission." Bill honked the horn a couple times out of elation. "My dad was a goddamn genius!"

Even Laura managed to smile. "Don't get your hopes up, Bill. Maybe the vial's only half full."

The wheels screeched as Bill careened into a space in front of the clinic and slammed on the brakes. He and Laura bolted up the walkway into the clinic. When they reached the small clinic lab, Bill threw open the freezer door. They both stared aghast. The freezer was empty.

28

"Are you sure it was in there?" Laura asked.

"Damn! It had to be." Bill slammed the freezer door shut. "Maybe I misread the label."

"If you did, then there would still be something there," Laura said. "Think," Laura faced him and grabbed both of his shoulders. "Where else could you have seen it?"

"Nowhere. It had to be there. I don't know. Maybe I'm losing my mind."

"So, we're back to where we started - waiting for outside help."

Bill nodded. Then his cell phone rang. He didn't recognize the number but answered anyway.

"Hello, Dr. Denton? I'm Dr. Anderson, Essex County Health Department Chief."

"Boy, am I glad to hear from you," Bill said. "Didn't you get my messages?"

"Uh, no. My secretary left me a note to call you but didn't mention the reason. I just received an emergency message on the CDC's internet-based Health Alert Network. All hell's broken loose since the President's press conference. How does Elizabethtown fit into all this?"

"It's where it all began."

"What? I'll be damned!" Dr. Anderson said. "Wait a second – that's not what they're broadcasting out of Washington, DC."

"If that's the case, then they're wrong."

"Can you fill me in?"

"I will," Bill said, "but right now I need you to get some people over here to help me track down who to vaccinate so we can be ready once we receive vaccine. How soon can you make it?"

"Give me an hour to round up a bunch of my nurses and techs. We've got to throw everything we can at this quickly, or it'll spin out of control."

"Too late. It already has," Bill said. "You've got my cell number. You know how bad cell service is in these parts, but hopefully you can reach me, when needed. Meet me at the Elizabethtown hospital emergency room as soon as you can. If I'm not there, I'll be at the high school. Oh, and bring any kind of medical supplies you can for vaccination: needles, alcohol, gauze pads and epinephrine for allergic reactions. Got any bifurcated needles?"

"You're kidding, right?"

"Just thought I'd ask. If the CDC doesn't send us any, we'll have to improvise. See you in a few." Bill hung up.

"Great news," Bill said to Laura. "At least we'll have a little help from the health department with this."

Bill's cell phone went off again. It was the ER. "There must be a patient over there," he said. "Let's go back. By the way, where the hell is Norm Phinney?"

"I have no idea. He should be at the hospital by now."

The two of them rushed out of the clinic and hopped back into the car. "Do me a favor," Bill said. "When we get back over there, see if you can find Norm. We could really use his help."

"Okay."

Bill's cell phone rang again, with a Washington, D.C. area code calling in. "It's Martinez. I hope he's got some good news." Bill answered the call while driving.

"What's the latest?" Bill asked.

"We're in crisis mode here," Martinez responded. "You were right. It *is* smallpox! As I told you, I saw that killer virus under the electron microscope with my own eyes, and my USAMRIID colleagues just confirmed it by PCR. They're sending a sample to CDC for culturing in order to test some possible countermeasures against it, but we're kind of grasping at straws. The only possible treatment we know of is intravenous cidofovir, which is toxic to the kidneys, and it's only been tested in monkey experiments to treat monkeypox, not smallpox. So, there are no guarantees it will work."

"Is there any way we could get some of that anyway? Right now, I've got nothing for my patients."

"Unlikely. I'm sorry. Any stocks of it are already being hoarded here in case any of the politicos get sick."

"What else is going on out there?"

"Since the President's press conference, the DC, Maryland, and Virginia health departments are working together. They've already tracked the locations where the Whitmans went during their Washington, DC school trip, and they've put the other children and parents who were in the group under quarantine at the Walter Reed Army Hospital in Washington, DC. A news bulletin has been sent out by the CDC to alert anyone who visited the Smithsonian or Congress during the same time to put themselves on home quarantine, check themselves for fever and to alert health authorities if they feel sick. We also just learned they visited the White House."

"Shit!" said Bill.

"Yeah," said Martinez. "The list is growing. The vaccine distribution plan has been activated."

"When do we get ours?" Bill asked.

"Bill, look out!" Laura yelled.

Bill slammed on his brakes barely in time to avoid rear-ending a car. He and Laura flew forward and the cell phone jettisoned out of Bill's hand onto the dashboard. Bill grabbed the phone.

"Martinez, are you there?"

"Yeah," Martinez answered. "What the hell was that?"

"Hold on, Martinez." Bill pulled over to the side of the road. "Sorry, man, we just missed a wreck by inches. Okay. So, when do we get our vaccine?"

"I don't know, Bill. I don't have direct control on where or how it's being used, but your town is definitely on the list."

"Ok. In the meantime, we'll do what we can to prepare. Don't leave us hanging, man. I've already had most of my hospital workers abandon ship and our sick patients continue to arrive."

"Roger that. I'll do what I can, and I'll keep you informed when I know something."

"Thank you." Bill hung up.

"So, what now?" Laura asked.

"Let's start by lining up whatever we can at the gym, so that if and when we receive vaccine, we'll be ready."

29

As they drove over to the school, Laura called the school principal. Shortly after they arrived at the parking lot, the principal pulled up in a beat-up station wagon. Bill and Laura got out of the car to meet him.

"Dr. Denton? Ms. Chen?" an unshaven, bald-headed man with the large nose greeted them. "I'm Beck Flagg. I came as soon as I could. Sorry I'm not more presentable. I'm not used to getting urgent calls this early in the morning."

"Understandable," Bill said. "We're just glad you're here."

"Follow me." He unlocked the door, and they followed the principal down the dark school corridors to the gymnasium. One by one, the principal flipped the gym's light switches on with a snap, and successive rows of white lights turned on, along with an electric buzzing sound. "Will this do?"

Bill surveyed the large gym, with its hardwood basketball court and one large bank of wooden bleachers.

"This will be perfect. Is there anyone you can call in to assist?"

"Yes. I've already reached several teachers. Many of the younger ones who have children were scared and refused, but the older cadre was quite enthusiastic. They ought to be trickling in soon."

Sure enough, within minutes, several gray-haired women came in. "Just tell us what you need," one said.

"Okay, if you have any tables you can set up, we'll need to first establish a one-way transit route. Patients can come in through that entrance," Bill pointed at the door on the right side of the bleachers. "The waiting area can be the first bank of bleachers. Then we'll need a line of screening tables and vaccination stations out here on the floor." He gestured to an area underneath one of the basketball baskets. "Then, once they've received vaccine, they can move to the left bank of bleachers to wait for a few minutes to ensure they're not having any problems. Finally, they'll exit out of that door." He pointed to the door on the left side of the bleachers. "Any questions?"

The ladies nodded their heads in agreement. "Let's hop to it," one of them said.

30

Norm Phinney turned off his television and nervously massaged the scar on his finger. The President's press conference confirmed Bill's suspicions: this had to be smallpox. Weeks ago, when Norm had first seen the frozen body, there was something about it that had seemed eerily familiar, but at the time, he ignored his suspicions. Now he remembered where he'd seen a photograph that looked similar. He pulled out a historical medical atlas and rifled quickly through the pages, tearing some of them in his haste. Sure enough, there it was: a picture of one of the ancient Egyptian pharaohs, Ramses V, who had died of smallpox. His mummified corpse was photographed in the Egyptian museum of antiquities in Cairo. The face had numerous slightly raised bumps on the surface of its shriveled, dry gray skin. The face and the skin lesions looked just like the frozen body's. If only he had thought to look for that picture earlier, the crisis might have never reached this stage.

He got up and paced the floor in his living room, periodically kicking at a hole in the threadbare green carpet in frustration.

"Shit!" There was no doubt in his mind: he was now a time bomb waiting to explode. Maybe he'd been able to get over a *Staph* finger infection, but he didn't think he'd fare so well with smallpox. He'd probably implanted the fucking virus from that frozen corpse right into his finger. Getting the disease by the respiratory route in the natural setting was one thing, but sticking a high concentration directly into his blood nearly guaranteed the virus would win.

He had no choice. If he was going to get sick, he wanted to at least have a fighting chance in a large hospital with a modern intensive care unit. Maybe they would find some new miracle drug to save him. He did a quick review of the medical literature and read about USAMRIID's experiments with a drug called cidofovir that had protected monkeys against similar viruses. Maybe he could get some, but he had to get out of town as quickly as possible before he came down with smallpox. There was no telling when or if the government might restrict travel. Every minute meant thousands more virus particles amplifying in his blood. He lumbered into his bedroom and threw as many clothes and toiletries as he could into two suitcases, stuffing them so full that he had to sit on them to get them closed before throwing them into the trunk of his car. Next, he grabbed a shovel from the garage and hurried into the back yard.

A couple years ago he had buried $3,000 in the woods behind his house for a rainy day, but he never anticipated needing it for something like this. It might come in handy if he needed to bribe someone to get cidofovir, especially if there was a run on healthcare facilities.

He sucked in deep breaths with every shovelful of dirt. Was he just out of shape or was he already getting sick? All the more reason to get moving. He heard a clink as the shovel hit the metal box. He dug a few more shovelfuls and then he threw the shovel on the ground. He reached into the hole and extracted a mud-smeared metal box full of money. He grabbed the box and moved as quickly as he could back to his car. With his foot jammed on the accelerator, he careened down the driveway so fast that he knocked over two garbage cans at the end of the driveway, launching them like missiles into his neighbor's yard.

31

Bill surveyed the gym. In a short half-hour, the teachers had set up multiple screening and vaccination tables and wrote signs to channel the patients through the different stations. They had also managed to scrounge a couple coolers from the football coach's office to keep the vaccine cool once it arrived. Bill put together a short screening form that would help to triage the patients into different categories. That way, if they needed to ration the vaccine supply, they could prioritize it first to those who already had a bona fide exposure to someone who was sick. After that, if there was vaccine left over, they could prioritize vaccine for healthcare personnel, young children, the elderly and other vulnerable populations.

"You ladies have done a great job," Laura said to the teachers. "Here's a contact sheet. Please place your name, address, and home phone number on it. If you have a cell phone, write that down as well. Now that everything is prepared, it's just a matter of waiting."

"Yes," said Bill. "We really appreciate your help. Go home now and rest but stay close to your telephones. Once we have more information on when the vaccine will arrive, we'll notify you to return."

Laura walked up to Principal Flagg. "Sir, thanks so much for your help in pulling everyone together."

"Happy to help," Flagg said. "It's times like these when a community shows its mettle. God help us. Give me a ring when you get the vaccine."

He left. Bill's cell phone rang.

"It's Martinez," he said.

"Bill," Martinez said, "how are you doing?"

"As best as can be imagined. Our vaccination setup is ready for whenever it comes. How are things on your end?"

"Not good. The President's declared a national emergency. CDC's hunting down contacts of the Whitmans, and they've received reports of smallpox from 15 states and 10 foreign countries."

"What the hell?" Bill said, his voice echoing in the gym.

"Yeah. Over the past several years, due to bioterrorism concerns, the U.S. manufactured enough smallpox vaccine to cover the nation. But now there are problems."

"Problems? What do you mean?" Bill started to feel tension rising in his gut. Laura gave him a worried look.

"The CDC is going to ration the vaccine. Your region was scheduled to receive doses from the national pharmaceutical stockpile. They were being flown up there along with a bunch of equipment on a 747, but now the governors of New York, Vermont, and New Hampshire are in a pissing contest on which state should get priority. One of the planes that was intended to loan vaccine to Canada has been hijacked."

"What the hell? Son of a bitch!"

"Three of the other vaccine stockpiles have been looted by armed thugs. Those locations are supposed to be secret, but obviously somebody had an inside connection. Vaccine's already being sold on the black market for $10,000 a pop. It's hell, Bill. It's hell. I'm sorry." Martinez's voice broke up as if he might cry.

"Are you telling me we're not getting any vaccine?"

There was no answer.

"Martinez?"

"I don't know, Bill." Martinez's voice was quiet. "This caught everyone totally by surprise. We've had all sorts of response drills over the last couple of years, but they never included someone looting our vaccine stockpiles. The FBI thinks some white supremacists and apocalyptic doomsday cults are behind it. The assault on the vaccine stores was very organized and must have been planned long ago with inside help. Where there *is* vaccine, people aren't waiting in line –

they're storming the barricades and having full-scale riots. Some people have been shot at distribution stations. I've never seen anything like it."

"Shit!" Bill swore.

"Yeah. The whole country's going to hell. The remaining doses in the stockpile are being hoarded by the federal government, with the first doses going to D.C. politicians and their family members. Then the military's getting its share, because the government's worried that North Korea or Russia might try something while we're pre-occupied.

"There are proposals to dilute what they have five-fold, but that will take time, and some vaccine will be lost in the process. Bifurcated needles that were stored with the vaccine are also missing. Congress and the press are pressuring the President to institute mass vaccination country wide. We had enough for that before, but with the significant losses already, there just isn't enough to go around."

"Can't they make some more?" Bill asked.

"Sure, but it takes time, and the Food and Drug Administration would never authorize its use without appropriate safety studies.

"Safety studies!" Bill screamed into the phone. "Who gives a shit about that if people are already dying?"

"Listen. It might not even get that far. There are rumors of explosions at some of the large pharmaceutical companies. Apparently, someone's been waiting for this opportunity to cripple us."

"What the hell?" Bill swore and kicked the bleachers. "So that's it, then? That's it?"

There was a pause on the line. "Yes. If I could do anything, I would."

"Sure, Martinez. I'm sure you would."

32

Bill hung up his phone and sat there for a moment, dazed. Then he filled Laura in on the pieces of the conversation she hadn't heard. Laura's shoulders slumped. Her hopeful facial expression turned into one of resignation.

"So, we're screwed," she said softly.

Bill let out a long sigh. He couldn't believe it. "Yes," he said quietly, and held her hand. Then he gave her a hug. He let go and looked at her drawn face and wiped off a tear.

"No use feeling sorry for ourselves, though," he said. "We can still make a difference and minimize this crisis as long as we can. We're the only ones who can. Let's go back to the hospital."

Laura nodded, as she dabbed her eyes with a tissue. Now that there was no vaccine coming, Bill really worried about what would happen to Laura and others who were exposed. The clock was ticking, and now there was very little he could do to slow or stop it.

On Main Street, blaring horns and screaming voices permeated the air.

"I've never seen anything like this," Bill remarked. Dozens of people crowded around the grocery store yelling.

Just as Bill pulled up to the four-way stop, he recognized the school's guidance counselor and gym teacher sprinting from the store with grocery bags in each arm. The store manager came running out with a shotgun and yelled "Stop thieves!" The sound of two shotgun blasts momentarily quieted the horns, but then they started up again. The two thieves escaped unscathed. As Bill drove away, the sound of shattering glass followed by an alarm made him turn his head. Someone had shattered one of the store's large front windowpanes, which started a mass looting.

"My God!" Laura said. "This is a full-scale panic!"

"If I didn't see it, I wouldn't believe it."

"When it's all over, will they be able to look at their neighbors again?"

"Maybe they won't *have* neighbors," Bill wondered aloud.

Bill and Laura entered the hospital through the back door and were greeted by shouting, screaming, and crying. The waiting room was filled with at least 30 people milling around and a line extending out the door and down the block, but no staff could be seen.

Dr. Brown rounded the corner carrying a clipboard with a patient record on it. He was looking more disheveled than when they left.

“How are you doing?” Bill asked.

“I’ve had better days. All the evaluation rooms are filled, and I’ve admitted two since you left, but they keep coming, as you can see. This is a masscal.”

“What do we do with them all?” Laura whispered.

“Good question,” Brown said. “I’ve just been working through them one at a time.”

“Yeah,” answered Bill. “We’re all making this up as we go along. Most of them probably aren’t sick, but they’re panicking after hearing the press conference.” The crowd mobbed him as he entered the waiting room.

“Dr. Denton, look at my child,” one woman tugged on his arm.

“Dr. Denton, help my baby,” another pleaded.

Bill struggled to get through the crowd to a spot where he could speak to everyone. He stood up on a table in a corner of the room. “Can I have your attention, please?” he called out and held up his hands. The voices diminished only slightly. He reached over and turned on an intercom switch by the triage nurse’s desk. “Please keep your voices down,” Bill’s voice projected throughout the room. Once the crowd quieted, he resumed. “You’ve probably seen the President’s press conference.” He reviewed what he knew about the press conference and provided some information about smallpox disease. “I know you’re scared, but please understand that most of you probably haven’t even been exposed to smallpox yet.” He hoped that what he said was true. “If you’re not sick, you shouldn’t be here. It increases your chances of being exposed to someone who *is* sick.”

The people began talking again. He didn’t know the best approach for the situation, but he couldn’t do much if he had to deal with such a mob.

“Dr. Brown, Nurse Chen, and I are the only ones here in the ER,” he gestured over to Laura and Joel, “and we have a single nurse on the ward as well as a laboratory technician. We will see *all* of you, one at a time, but we need your cooperation, because we can’t help those who are really ill if we have to see people who are just afraid. If you don’t have a fever, then you don’t have smallpox. It’s as simple as that. Raise your hand if you have a fever.” Only five people raised their hands. The others around them immediately moved away nervously. “Okay – I need all five of you to go with Ms. Chen so she can take your vital signs.” The five people got up and moved toward Laura.

“Now,” Bill said, “I don’t have any smallpox vaccine yet. We’re trying to get some. If you’re not sick, the best thing you can do is go home. Once we get the vaccine, we’ll make an announcement all over town about how you can get it.”

This seemed to satisfy some of them. A few of them got up to leave.

“Before you go,” said Bill, “I want to make sure I get your name, address, and phone number.”

Bill recognized many of them from his childhood or from seeing them in the clinic, but he didn’t want to rely on just his memory to track them down. He passed around a sign-in roster. Then he walked over to the nurse’s station to see how Laura was doing. She just finished getting vital signs on the last of the five patients.

“What have you got?” he asked.

“Only two of them have fevers, after all.” She

indicated the exam rooms where she'd placed those patients.

Bill grabbed their charts. "Okay, Joel and I will divide them up and see them one at a time. Keep the peace out here."

"Roger," Laura said.

"Oh" – Bill turned back to her – "and slap on an N95 mask again. We can always hope we haven't been exposed yet, and the less exposure we have, the lower our chances of getting infected."

Laura opened a drawer near her, took a mask, and handed another to Bill. Bill put it on and entered the exam room.

He saw two patients back-to-back. Both had moderate fevers and rashes in the early stages. One had done some carpentry work in the Whitmans' home a couple weeks earlier. The other worked in the school cafeteria. The other three patients that Dr. Brown saw didn't have a fever or any definite exposure to the construction workers or their children, and they admitted they came to the ER simply out of fear. Bill made sure to get their names, phone numbers, and addresses before they left so they could be tracked down later.

Bill and Joel assessed the remaining patients one by one. Fortunately, most were not ill, but more kept coming. The hours dragged on. Eventually, the sun came up and morning changed to afternoon. Bill feared that the hospital would turn out to be the central area for disease spread, so Laura made a sign for the ER entrance to indicate that only patients with fevers or serious injuries would be seen – all others were warned to stay away. The sign seemed to do the trick. Eventually the flow of patients ebbed.

After clearing out his last patient at 3:00 p.m., Bill collapsed on a couch in the waiting room, exhausted. Joel was seeing his last patient in an exam room. "You know," Bill said to Laura, while resting his feet on a chair, "we make a damn good team."

Laura sat down next to him and took off her mask. "I hope we live through this so we can do it again."

"I'm all for that. By the way, I'm starving. You want something from the vending machine? Have you eaten anything today?"

"No. I've been so busy, I forgot all about food. I guess I'll have a bag of chips."

Bill walked down the deserted hallway to a small room with vending machines. The money clinked its way through the machine before the lights on the number pad lit up. He punched in the numbers for a candy bar, potato chips, and soda and waited for the familiar thud as they fell into the receptacle.

"Bill," Laura yelled, "come here, STAT!"

Bill ran down the hallway into the waiting room. Henry O'Donnell was pushing his wife in a wheelchair through the front door. Her face was flushed, and she mumbled while turning her head back and forth.

"There," Bill said, pointing across the ER. "Put her in room one." Laura wheeled her in and the mayor followed. "What happened?" Bill asked.

"She had a bad headache last night. I let her sleep in today, thinking it was one of her migraines, but she never woke up. This afternoon when I checked on her she was babbling - didn't even recognize me."

Bill yanked on some gloves and a mask and then felt her forehead. "She's burning up. Laura, get some vital signs – and put your mask back on!"

They lifted Mrs. O'Donnell onto the exam table where Bill inspected her closely. She mumbled incoherently. Small bumps had developed on her face and hands; she breathed rapidly, and her heart raced. Bill had flashbacks of Felicia Jamison and Jeremy Whitman.

"Temp's 105," said Laura. "Respiratory rate's 30 and pulse is 120. BP's 110/70."

"Is she gonna be okay?" Henry asked.

Bill pulled Henry to the side of the room and spoke quietly. "She's very ill. She's probably got smallpox."

"Damn!" Henry swore.

"*Now* do you believe me?" Bill asked. "This *is* smallpox – it's been confirmed in Washington, DC. Go out to the waiting room. I'll come get you as soon as I've finished my exam."

"Doc, what I said before, I –"

"Don't bother to apologize, Henry. Just do as I ask."

Henry left the room with his shoulders slumped and his head bowed.

"Okay, let's get an IV in her," Bill said. Laura handed him an intravenous catheter and prepared an IV fluid bag. Bill tied a tourniquet on the woman's arm and swabbed it with an alcohol pad. He slapped the arm a couple times to make the veins stand out, then inserted a needle into a prominent vein until he saw a flash of blood in the syringe indicating he was in the right spot. The catheter advanced easily over the needle into the vein. Once attached to the catheter, the IV bag began running fluid into the woman's vein. As he taped the catheter onto her arm to hold it in place, Bill noticed a bandage on the woman's upper outer arm, near her shoulder. Curious, he removed the bandage, revealing some soiling and blood on the bandage. There was an array of multiple tiny red spots in a circular pattern about the size of a dime on her skin. "Laura, check this out."

Laura came over to Bill's side of the exam table. He pointed out the spots. "What do you make of that?"

"Looks like she's been stuck with a needle – multiple times."

"That's what I thought," said Bill.

"How fast do you want the IV fluid to run in?" Laura asked.

"Give her a 500 ml bolus over about 20 minutes and then change it to 125 mls per hour."

"Got it," Laura said as she adjusted the IV fluid dial.

Bill continued to stare at the needle marks. "Damn!" He suddenly realized it could only mean one thing. "When does someone get stuck with a needle just on the surface of their skin multiple times?"

Laura stopped what she was doing. She bent down and looked closely at the woman's arm again. "I don't know."

"Sure you do," said Bill, frowning. "Smallpox vaccine!"

"What? That means she's just been vaccinated. How?"

"I'm not sure, but I've got a hunch. That *bastard*!" Bill swore and kicked the wall. "The missing vaccine vial!"

"Oh my God! How else?"

"How else, indeed! Wait here." He put his finger to his lips. "Play along with me and don't say anything." Bill stuck his head out the door. "Henry, could you come in here?"

Henry entered a moment later.

"Henry, we should keep your wife in the hospital for now, so we can at least continue to give her fluids. Unfortunately, I don't have any specific treatment for her."

Henry hung his head. "I understand. Listen doc, I'm sorry for the way I behaved."

"I told you I don't need an apology. What I need is an explanation, though." Bill pointed at the woman's arm. "Do you know what happened there?"

"I – I don't know," Henry said, his face turning red as he averted Bill's gaze.

"Hmm," Bill said. "If I had to guess, it looks like someone gave her the smallpox vaccine."

"No, I…"

"Where did you get it, Henry?"

"I didn't…"

"Damn you!" Bill shoved Henry's heavy frame up against the wall. "You think I'm an idiot? Someone vaccinated her. Who? Where's the vaccine?"

"I don't have it," Henry answered.

Bill grabbed Henry's left arm and tore down the sleeve from the shoulder seam. On the upper outer part of the mayor's arm was a bandage, which Bill tore off. He saw the same markings.

"You selfish bastard. Where'd you get the vaccine? What have you done with it?"

Henry slumped to the ground. "Rosemary found it when she worked for your father. She has it."

"She stole it from the clinic?" Bill asked. "Where is she?"

"She's at my house. She's sick too."

"Come on, Laura," Bill said. "Let's get that vaccine." Laura and Bill bounded to the hospital exit.

"It's too late," Henry called after them.

Bill and Laura stopped. "What are you talking about?" Bill asked.

"I think she sold it."

33

The noise of the town faded as Bill drove toward Henry's home in a more remote area on the side of Cobble Hill. He pulled the car up Henry's driveway. The house was dark except for the porch light.

"You stay here," Bill said to Laura.

"Good luck," Laura responded, patting him on the arm.

Bill walked cautiously up to the house and onto the porch. The place was quiet. He could see through the kitchen window that some of the interior lights were on. He banged on the door. No response. He banged again. Nothing. He turned the handle, which wasn't locked and tentatively entered the kitchen.

"Rosemary?" he called, "it's Dr. Denton."

He heard no response. He started to leave the kitchen heading toward the living room.

"What do you want?" Rosemary said, as she emerged from the hallway on the other side of the kitchen. Her voice was hoarse and weak.

"You have something I need," Bill said. "Where's the vaccine?"

"What vaccine? I don't know what you're talking about."

"Don't play games with me. People are dying, and Henry told me you have it. I know you stole it from the clinic."

Rosemary hesitated. She didn't look well. Her face was flushed, and her eyes were red and watery. Small vesicles were visible around her face.

"That bastard," Rosemary swore, "I told him to keep his mouth shut."

"Hand it over. I need it to quell the outbreak."

"You know what it's worth, doctor? Someone in

Keene Valley offered me $15,000 for this vial. Why should I give it up? I found it."

"Because you're a nurse, Rosemary. This isn't like you."

"Oh yeah, easy for you to say. You got to escape this town. I'm stuck here. This is my ticket out."

"Are you kidding? There's no way out, Rosemary. We're all trapped. You can help me to save some others. Where is it?" Bill suspected that Rosemary would want to keep the vaccine cool while she was negotiating a sale. He lunged for the refrigerator and threw open the door. He caught a glimpse of the vial on the top shelf of the refrigerator and grabbed it. Rosemary rammed into Bill's side, knocking him to the floor. She jumped on top of him and pummeled him with her fists and scratched his face. As they struggled, Bill was surprised by how strong she was, even while sick. Rosemary pulled on his arm, while trying to grab the vial out of his hand. Bill successfully pushed her away with his other hand and gave her a swift kick. She fell back and hit her head against the stove. Bill crawled away from her reach, the vial still in his hand.

"Rosemary, you're infected, I can see that. Come with me to the hospital so I can evaluate you."

"Liar. It's just a cold."

"I can already see the rash forming, Rosemary. It's obvious. Just look in the mirror. Come with me."

"No way."

"Suit yourself," Bill said. He stood up and turned toward the door to leave.

"Bastard," Rosemary said as she grabbed a mop and swung it against Bill's arm. The force of the mop wrenched Bill's arm backwards, causing him to release the vial. He watched in horror as the vial flew from his hand. As if in slow motion, the vial bounced once off the tile floor and shattered as it hit the floor a second time. Bill stood there, staring at the shards of glass strewn about the floor, mixed in with the splashed contents of the vial.

"I - I'm...sorry," Rosemary said, "I – I didn't realize..." her voice faded to a whisper.

Bill didn't know what to say. In an instant, his hope for the town was shattered, along with the vial. He silently turned and walked out the door.

"Dr. Denton," Rosemary called after him. "Don't go. Don't leave me here."

Bill stepped off the porch and got back into the car. "How did you get those scratches on your face?" Laura asked.

"The vial's gone," Bill said, ignoring her question. "Let's go back to the hospital."

34

Bill's cell phone rang.

"Martinez?"

"Hi Bill. What's the latest there?"

"It's a long story, but we found a single vial of smallpox vaccine that my father had save, but it has been destroyed. What about you?"

"Oh? What? I'm really sorry to hear that. The President has just declared martial law. The Feds are pissed because some governors closed their state borders already without consulting them, which has stymied interstate transit. Our national borders are also closed. Public gatherings are being restricted, and a national curfew's been instituted. The stock market's crashed. No other countries will allow our planes to land, so the skies are a mess."

"Tell me some good news, Martinez."

"I don't have any. The National Guard's been activated in several states on the East Coast to maintain order, including New York. There have been some key regions targeted for mass quarantine. Your town is one of them."

"What? You mean they're going to just cut us off? Are we on our own?"

"I hope not, Bill. They're hoping the epidemic will burn itself out if certain places are isolated. The National Guard's probably already shut down the exits out of your valley. If not, I'd get out while you can…" The phone cut off.

"Martinez? Martinez!" Bill yelled into the phone. He checked the battery, which was still working. He tried to call Martinez back repeatedly, but received a busy signal at first, then no signal at all. He shut off the phone.

35

Bill and Laura rushed back through the emergency room. Bill grabbed Henry by the arm and yelled in his face. "You bastard. The vial's been destroyed. Now we're completely screwed. Don't you give a shit about anyone?"

"I was scared," Henry protested. "I didn't know what to do. How could I maintain order if I was sick?"

"Order? What the hell are you talking about? It's too late for that. You destroyed our only chance. The hospital staff's deserted and the town's in shambles."

Laura pulled on Bill's arm. "He's not worth your time and energy. If anyone survives this, they'll judge him accordingly."

"You're right." Bill let go of Henry's arm.

Moments later, Dr. Brown rushed in. "A woman just drove up outside. She's got someone bleeding in the back of her car!"

Dr. Brown and Laura rushed outside, followed by Bill. Bill recognized Nettie emerging from her rattling, beat-up brown Plymouth, which spewed thick gray exhaust.

"What happened?" Bill asked her as he approached the car.

"There's a terrible traffic jam of cars trying to get out of the valley. This fellow smacked his car near the Post Office during the mad dash."

Bill peered into the back seat. "Shit! It's Norm! Joel, get me a stretcher and a neck collar! STAT!"

Dr. Brown disappeared back into the hospital and reappeared with a stretcher, a C-collar, and other equipment. Bill put gloves on and secured the collar around Norm's neck, and Laura helped him carefully extract Norm from the back seat. Bill made a quick trauma survey. Norm was unconscious and bleeding from his mouth and nose. Bill stemmed some of the bleeding with gauze. Norm had sustained a large bruise on his left cheek. Otherwise, his vital signs were stable, and he didn't appear to have any broken bones or abdominal injuries. "Let's get him inside," Bill said.

They wheeled Norm into the emergency room, then Bill performed a secondary examination to ensure he hadn't missed anything life-threatening. Everything appeared normal except for Norm's loss of consciousness. Bill didn't have a CT scanner to assess for internal head injuries, but what he could perform of a neurologic exam did not show any focal abnormalities, but he couldn't be sure until Norm awakened. He stopped Norm's nosebleed with some nasal packing, then he sutured a gash in Norm's mouth while quizzing Nettie.

"It's horrible," Nettie said. "Everyone's trying to escape, but the National Guard's already shut off the pass just south of town. They even shot old man Warner when he tried to run the roadblock." Nettie began to weep. "He's dead," she sobbed.

"See?" Henry piped in from across the room. "Even the National Guard's scared. Can't blame them. We haven't seen the likes of this since polio when I was a kid.

"Henry," Bill said, momentarily turning his attention away from assessing Norm. "Listen. There's not much you can do here, but you can still help out. I need you to take charge. Round up your sheriff and deputies. Make them establish a security perimeter around the central town to stop the looting. Get someone to control traffic on Main Street and send some others down to the roadblock to establish order. Establish a curfew and start patrolling the neighborhood. You need to keep everyone from panicking."

Henry appeared to mull this over. Then he walked slowly over to the nurse's station and played with the telephone. A few minutes later he returned.

"Phones are out. Doc. Is she gonna make it?" He began sobbing heavily.

Laura took him aside and consoled him until he

calmed down.

"She's stable now," Bill said. "but there's not much I can do but wait and watch. I promise I'll take care of her as if she were my own mother."

Henry seemed to be reassured. "Thanks, Doc, but I can't leave."

"What? Henry," Bill said, "this is crazy. You're in charge. Go take charge."

Henry shook his head. "I can't leave while my wife is sick."

"Shit," Bill swore, as he thought how he could maintain order without Henry. Then he got an idea.

"Henry, you know Jed Thorton, the lead construction worker, right?"

Henry nodded.

"He's a retired Army sergeant major. Who better to help establish some order? I need you to do just one thing for me. Drive out to his house and bring him here. Please, Henry. Can you at least do that?"

Henry wiped his tears with his sleeve and sat there for a minute. "Ok. I'll go find Jed and see if he'll come back with me."

"Not *if* Henry. Tell him that *Major Denton* has ordered him to come here immediately."

Henry got up and left.

Several other patients entered the waiting room and Dr. Brown took care of them.

Bill resumed attending to Norm in one of the emergency room bays. Bill drew blood while Laura ran an EKG and Nettie looked on. As Bill inserted an IV into Norm's hand, Laura cleaned some blood off Norm's other hand.

"Did you see this scar on Norm's finger?" Laura asked.

"Yeah," Bill said. He finished putting the IV in and hung a bag of IV fluid before he turned his attention to where Laura was pointing. "Remember? I told you that Norm cut himself a couple weeks ago."

"Oh, yeah. I remember now." Laura resumed cleaning the blood off Norm. "But wait a second," she burst out suddenly. "Norm had contact with that frozen body the same day as those construction workers, right?"

"Yeah."

"Then why doesn't *he* have smallpox?" Laura asked.

"We already talked about this. He used to work with viruses. He was probably vaccinated."

Laura nodded. "Maybe…but check out his arms. I don't find a vaccine scar anywhere."

Bill examined Norm's upper arms closely. "You're right. I don't see any scars, but sometimes the scars can be small."

"Maybe, but what if he didn't get vaccinated? That would still beg the question," Laura said, "why didn't he get smallpox yet?"

"I don't know."

"We need him to wake up so we can ask him," said Laura.

"Wait," said Bill, his voice rising in pitch from excitement. "Maybe he *was* vaccinated after all."

"What do you mean?"

"I just realized something. The virus that causes smallpox is the Variola virus. The smallpox vaccine uses a different virus, the Vaccinia virus, to protect us. Vaccinia is a close cousin to Variola. It is similar enough to provide protection, but it's not as dangerous as smallpox virus."

"What's your point?" asked Laura.

"My point is: if someone gets a direct inoculation in their skin with smallpox virus, it can have the same effect as vaccination. That's probably what happened to Norm when he cut his finger. Look," he said, while holding up Norm's finger, "doesn't that look like a smallpox vaccine scar?"

"Damn!" Laura slapped her hand on the side of the exam table. "It *does*. I didn't think of that because it's in a different location than where I'm used to seeing it."

"So," Bill said, "if Norm was protected by his cut, why couldn't someone else be protected in the same way? In fact, that's exactly what some ancient cultures did before they had a vaccine. They ground up smallpox scabs and put them on an open wound. It was called variolation."

"You're right," Laura said. "I'd forgotten that. It's *possible* to confer protection against smallpox, by actually using the smallpox virus to inoculate the skin. But it's risky."

"Yes," Bill said. "So, it is a bit ironic, but you could use the deadly smallpox virus in a manner that prevents the same deadly disease – smallpox. But doing so has risks. Not everyone would be protected - some people could actually get smallpox."

"True, but fewer than if they're infected the usual way, through their nose or mouth. I seem to recall that using variolation caused death in around 1-3%."

"Yes, but that compares with a 30% death rate from smallpox without variolation."

Bill sat down next to Norm's gurney. "I can't believe this. The solution to our problem has been staring us in the face all along. We can use some of the smallpox virus from one of our victims to inoculate the town."

"Why not?" Laura said. "There's a risk, obviously, for transmitting other infections, like hepatitis or HIV, since you'll be taking fluid and pus from someone for use on others, but without the usual rigorous safety testing."

"Yeah," Bill said, "but we can minimize that risk by taking the virus from someone we know didn't have those infections."

"Who?"

Bill thought for a moment. "My father."

"What? No."

"Hear me out," Bill said. "I know my dad's medical history, and he was as healthy as a horse until he had that stroke. Using variolation is better than just sitting here doing nothing. Besides, anyone in this town who has been vaccinated against smallpox before may have some residual immunity, so the 1-3% rate of smallpox occurring and causing death after variolation may be lower. We may lose some people, but we're going to lose a lot more if we don't do anything. We can try and minimize risk, though by targeting only those with a definite exposure to someone already sick. Then we can create herd immunity to block transmission to those who are susceptible."

"Works for me," Laura said.

The mayor returned with Jed Thorton in tow.

Jed walked up to Bill and snapped a quick salute. "Sergeant Major Thorton reporting for duty, sir. How can I help?"

Bill saluted back, then he described the situation. "I need you to take charge of the town in place of the mayor. Work with the sheriff to establish some order. Henry can introduce you to the sheriff."

"Roger that. Mayor O'Donnell," Jed said, "get your ass moving."

Henry obediently stood up and followed Jed out the door.

"Okay," said Bill. "Once they get a handle on things, we can enlist the sheriff's help to keep people at home to minimize exposures. That's where Jed could really help us. We can also issue masks and gloves to the family members of smallpox victims. With nothing else to go on, it's time to go back to basics: good old-fashioned quarantine, hand-washing, and respiratory protection. We've got no time to lose. Nettie!" Bill turned to her. "I need your help to stay here and watch over Norm and the mayor's wife. Be very careful to use a mask whenever you go in Mrs. O'Donnell's room."

"Dear," Nettie said, patting Bill's arm, "I've lived through measles, whooping cough, and polio. You think I'm scared of a little smallpox? It's been a while since I took care of my father, but helping patients will come back to me pretty quick."

"You're wonderful," Bill said. "Even so, we'll make sure to inoculate you as well. Dr. Brown is here, too, so he can help you out, if needed."

Bill and Laura set to work collecting sterile needles, alcohol, gauze pads, and bandages. Bill then rushed down to the morgue and donned a gown, gloves, and a mask. He pulled out the drawer holding his father and paused for a moment observing his father's peaceful, gray body. Seeing him again in this state caused a new wave of emotion. "Focus," he said to himself, as he suppressed a sob.

"You figured it out, Dad. Don't worry. It won't be in vain. We're going to lick this thing."

He then carefully punctured numerous vesicles on his father's hands and arms. As the fluid oozed out of the vesicles, Bill collected it in a sterile vial. He then mixed the vesicle fluid with some normal saline to create a vaccine solution. By diluting the concentration of virus in the vial he hoped to make the solution safer. He held the clear vial up to the light. In that small vial, there were probably millions of tiny smallpox virus particles floating in the solution. They held the key to saving the town. Bill closed the drawer and ran back upstairs to meet with Laura.

"It's only appropriate to do this on ourselves before we try it on others," Bill said. "I'll go first – you can inoculate me."

"Okay," Laura said. "This is kind of scary without bifurcated needles."

"I know," Bill said, "but we'll just have to use straight needles usually used for blood draws instead and hope that the amount at the tip of the needle is just enough to provide protection without killing us."

"This isn't without precedent, you know," Laura said, "medical researchers experimenting on themselves. I only hope it works."

Laura put on gloves and then inoculated Bill with

fluid and multiple pinpricks on his arm, and then she covered the area with a bandage. Bill in turn inoculated Laura and then Nettie after they returned to the hospital.

"Okay," said Bill, "with the roadblock, the county health department people will never get here, and I've got no easy way to bring the teachers back to the gym, so we're going to have to do mass vaccination ourselves, house – by – house. Nettie, unfortunately, it looks like we don't have cell service anymore. We'll come back periodically for an update on the patients."

36

Bill and Laura picked up a town map from the sheriff's office. An eerie stillness had settled over the town. No one was outside now and the cars had disappeared.

"Jed must have finally mobilized the sheriff and his deputies," Bill said to Laura, as he saw some of them patrolling various street corners throughout the town. "I'm glad we convinced the sheriff to have all of his deputies inoculated, since they are at high risk." He had also issued the sheriff enough masks to cover his team.

Bill and Laura methodically stopped at each house, quizzed the inhabitants about their possible contacts, and variolated those associated with the school or with exposure risk to the construction workers' families. One by one, Laura checked the houses off on the map. By the time they made the rounds to about half of the houses, they counted 10 people who were already sick. All those victims' family members gladly accepted variolation. Another quarter of some lower-risk people insisted on getting it, too. Bill even convinced some of the nurses, who had fled the hospital, to return and assist Nettie once they had been variolated.

The sun had set by the time Bill drove into one of the local gas stations, where his patient, Walt Richards and his family lived. "Wait here," he said, and left Laura in the car while he went to check inside.

The bell attached to the door rang as Bill entered the deserted station. A single bulb in the middle of the ceiling cast an eerie yellow haze around the office where spare automobile parts were scattered. Grease coated every piece of equipment, from the soda machine to the cash register, and the smell of whiskey permeated the air.

"Walt?" Bill called, his voice echoing in the empty garage next to the office. Not hearing an answer, Bill turned to leave. As he grabbed the door handle, he heard a shuffle behind him.

"Hooollldddd it!"

Bill froze. He recognized Walt's Adirondack drawl, but his words slurred together - probably related to the whiskey odor.

In the grimy plexi-glass window in front of him, Bill could barely see Walt's swaying form behind him and the shotgun pointed at his head. He didn't dare move, practically shivering from fear and his breath came in short gasps. Not wanting to show his fear, he tried to keep his voice steady by using short sentences.

"Walt, what is it? What do you want?"

"Haven't you heard? There's disease in this here town. I don't want you bringin' me disease. Ya hear?"

"Of course," Bill replied, his voice now pleading. "Walt, you know me. I'm not sick. I wouldn't come here if I were sick."

"Oh yeah?"

"Yes, Walt, I'm here to help you. You and your family."

"You stay away from us!"

Bill realized it was pointless to try and reason with the man. While keeping his head steady, his eyes darted around, frantically searching for a weapon. The slightest movement could be his last. He saw nothing within easy reach.

"If you think I'm diseased, then let me go. If I'm sick, the longer you keep me here, the greater your chances of getting it." Bill hoped Walt was digesting the information. If he kept talking, keeping Walt off guard, he might have the opportunity to gain the upper hand. "If you shoot me, then my blood would contaminate you."

None of what Bill said seemed to help. "Walt! I'm your doctor. I would never do anything to harm you. If you don't want me here, then let me go so I can help others."

"Ain't good enough, Doc. Tell that to the undertaker."

Walt pulled back the hammer on the shotgun.

Bill dove for the floor at the same time as he spun around, kicking the shotgun muzzle upward. He felt the shock wave from the shotgun as it blasted out the window above his head. Walt was momentarily knocked back by the recoil from the shotgun and Bill's kick. He fell backward against the counter, but he grabbed another shell to reload the weapon. Bill knocked the shotgun barrel upwards again and the second blast peppered the ceiling. Bill then dove for Walt's midsection, just as another figure leaped into the room, hitting Walt squarely in the shoulders. The force of the two knocked Walt back into the counter again. Bill looked up in time to see Laura kick Walt square in the stomach, causing him to bend forward. Next she gave him a swift knee to his chin, which made him sprawl backward and onto the floor. Meanwhile, Bill grabbed the shotgun from Walt, who by now was flat on his back on the floor with Laura standing menacingly over him.

Bill trained the shotgun on Walt, but he lost his balance and collapsed backward against what was left of the door. All the while, though, he kept the shotgun pointed at Walt. Walt made a couple attempts to get up again, but Laura quickly whacked him until he gave up.

"Okay, Walt," Bill said, "don't piss me off again. We came here to help you." With Walt now subdued, Bill tried to explain to him what they were doing. "Your kids go to school with two of the victims, Jeremy Whitman and Felicia Jamison. They're at high risk, Walt. Let us inoculate them."

"Go to hell!" Walt swore.

After a few more attempts to reason with Walt, Bill and Laura gave up and left the gas station, but they made sure to bring the shotgun with them. As they were getting back in the car, Walt's wife came running out of the shop.

"Doctor Denton. Don't go. Please help us." Walt and his wife then proceeded to have an argument, which she eventually won. "Don't be a drunken old fool," she said to

Walt. She brought her four kids out of the house and lined them up for Laura to variolate.

Once all kids were taken care of, Bill and Laura got back into the car and drove on to the next house.

"Where did you learn to move like that?" Bill asked. "I was impressed. You saved my life."

"Gotta know how to protect yourself when you live in New York City. I'm sure you'll think of a way to make it up to me." She patted his hand and grinned.

"Now I've had two people pull shotguns on me today – things can only get better."

After visiting a couple more houses, they stopped by the hospital to check up on Nettie, Dr. Brown, and their patients. About a quarter of the hospital staff had now returned. Norm had recovered consciousness, but he still had some residual amnesia. Bill walked into the room to check on the mayor's wife. She didn't look good. Multiple skin lesions had blossomed and coalesced into pockets of pus on her face and hands. She writhed constantly and moaned from the pain. Bill prescribed some morphine, which helped to calm her down for now.

"We have to let someone outside town know what we're doing." Bill said to Laura. "Others could benefit if they don't have enough vaccine." Bill tried to call Martinez again, but the line was still dead. He walked into Norm's room. "Norm, if the phone lines are down, is there any way to send an email? Or a text message?"

"No," said Norm. "Cell phones still feed into the local land lines. You could always try a short-wave radio, but I don't know anyone who's got one."

"Great. I guess there's nothing we can do until the phone lines come back up. I'll resume variolating."

This time Laura recruited two nurses to help, after she demonstrated the proper technique. All four of them then headed for the door.

"Wait!" Norm called after them. "If you had a

satellite hook-up, that would by-pass the local phone lines."

"You have one?"

"No. Sorry."

"Great! If *you* don't have one, I doubt anyone else would."

"Wait!" Laura grabbed Bill's arm. "You mean for the Internet? Remember your patient, Lillian Johnson? The librarian?"

"Uh huh," Bill grunted.

"I'm almost positive she said the library's got a satellite hook-up for its Internet."

"Wow," said Bill, "let's get over there then." Bill showed the two other nurses the map and instructed them where to resume the inoculations from where he and Laura had left off. "We'll catch up with you as soon as we can send off an email."

Bill sped over to the library. Rather than try to find Mrs. Johnson this time, Bill decided to break in. All was quiet in the immediate vicinity, although horns and sirens sounded in the distance, along with an occasional bang from gunfire. A grove of trees stood next to the library, shielding it from any houses within potential viewing distance. Bill walked up to the window and peered in. The room was dark, except for the flicker of a computer screensaver to his left. Hopefully that would be his connection. The window didn't yield to his attempts to jimmy it, so he picked up a rock the size of his fist and smashed the glass. He then took off his shirt, rolled it up around his hand and arm as he brushed the broken glass off the sill before unlocking and pushing up the window. He climbed in. The inside smelled a bit musty. It took a moment for his eyes to adjust to the dark. He stepped forward, but froze, feeling a tug on his right shoulder. Turning his head slowly, he jumped when he realized he was looking straight into the face of a deer trophy.

With a sigh of relief, he turned back to the window. "Go around front," he said to Laura. "I'll let you in there."

Once Laura was inside, Bill locked the door again and Laura led him to the computer she'd used previously for Internet access.

"I hope this password works," said Laura. "Lillian gave it to me early this morning. Cross your fingers."

Bill unconsciously crossed his fingers while Laura typed into the keyboard.

"We're in," she said. "It *must* be a satellite hookup."

"Great!" said Bill. They gave each other a high five as they traded seats. "Let me see if Martinez has his ears on." Bill searched his pocket and found Martinez's email address. He typed in the address and then wrote a note:

Martinez, are you there? Our phone lines are down. We're unable to get any info. What's the latest? --Bill

Bill sent the message. At least five minutes passed without any response.

"Well," Bill said, "even if he's not there, I can at least leave him a message about our variolation campaign." He proceeded to type.

Martinez – since there's no vaccine coming, we began inoculating those at highest risk with fluid from smallpox vesicles – like the ancient practice of variolation. If there is a shortage of vaccine elsewhere, it's an option worth considering. Bill clicked on the send button.

Another few minutes passed.

"He must not be there," Laura said.

"You're right" Bill guided the arrow on the computer screen to the *close* button. As he was about to click on it, a *NEW MESSAGE* notice flashed on the computer screen.

"It's Martinez!" They both cheered.

Bill, glad to know you're still with us. I was getting worried about you when our conversation got cut off. The phone and cell lines are out in pockets all over the country due to the heavy call volume. We have some of the few lines that are still intact. To make matters worse, there have also been different Internet viruses unleashed. I'm amazed you were able to send me a message.

They're trolling for vaccine anywhere they can find it. The northeast is in mayhem. The National Guard's been activated all across the U.S. to maintain order. This is having a chain reaction all across the world. In Europe they're quarantining any American who stepped off a plane in the last two weeks, unless they can show proof of smallpox vaccine. But who could, even if they had received it? It's not even on the yellow international shot card anymore! Needless to say, the public health guys are completely overwhelmed. They now have armed guards at all vaccine stations, but vaccine continues to be ripped off, and some more people have been shot trying to steal it. The price of vaccine on the black market's now up to $100,000.

"Wow!" Bill said. He responded by typing: *Any more cases of smallpox since the Whitmans? We've counted 10 here so far.*

Bill clicked on *SEND*.

Moments later, another message appeared.

I've heard of cases in a dozen major cities in Europe, including Paris and Frankfurt, just to name a few. There are reports of outbreaks in Africa – they don't know whether those are from monkeypox, smallpox, or even chickenpox, because lots of misinformation is being spread on the Internet. The anti-vaccine groups are in rare form. That Whitman girl exposed a hell of a lot of people during her visit to Washington, DC. A preliminary report I saw from the airline estimated that of the 150 people on board, at least half of them subsequently traveled out of the country.

We're at the point where the politicians won't let us target the main individuals who have been exposed, because they want control of the vaccine. What little vaccine we have is being wasted on people not really at risk, but who have political influence.

Bill typed: *How quickly could they crank out more vaccine?*

Martinez responded: *With some of the major manufacturers being bombed, cranking up production could take months, if not years. Newer lots of vaccine have only been tested in small numbers of people so far, so the pharmaceutical companies and the FDA are reluctant to release them. The President has railroaded a new vaccine indemnity bill through Congress, but the pharmaceutical companies are still concerned about being sued. Who can blame them after the swine flu vaccine fiasco back in the 70s? Don't look for any more vaccine anytime soon.*

Bill turned toward Laura, who was reading over his shoulder. "Good thing we're doing what we're doing."

"Yeah," she said. "We'd be sunk otherwise."

Is the CDC going to send anyone here? Bill clicked on *SEND*.

Martinez responded: *Right now, they're too overwhelmed elsewhere to bother with your town. Since it's quarantined, that takes care of the problem for now. Eventually someone might make it there - more likely someone from the FBI, trying to track down a terrorist.*

"Damn!" Bill swore. "I told him this wasn't from terrorism."

He typed: *Martinez, I told you this wasn't bioterrorism. If you send someone up here to get a lab sample from the frozen body, you could have USAMRIID or CDC do a DNA fingerprint on the virus and show that it's the same as the other victims. That would prove how this whole fiasco originated.*

Bill clicked on the *SEND* button. A moment later, a dialogue box appeared on the screen: *Your connection has been interrupted.*

"Shit! He might not get my last message."

"That figures," said Laura.

Bill attempted to log on several more times but couldn't re-establish the connection.

"Looks like nothing's changed – we're still on our

own," Bill said. "Let's catch up with the others and continue our variolation strategy."

As they headed toward the door, Bill heard some angry voices out front. It sounded like a gang of teenagers. Before he could open the door, one of the front windows shattered, and a Molotov cocktail flew in and exploded on the floor, sending glass shards and flames everywhere. Bill and Laura ducked just in time and hit the floor behind one of the book stacks. Bill grabbed Laura's hand, and they crawled to the back window where Bill had entered and climbed out, just as the library behind them was consumed by flames.

37

Fortunately, the teenagers had left by the time Bill and Laura rounded the building, and their car was still intact, but the library inferno crackled and spat as the wooden building went up in flames in minutes like an out-of-control wildfire. They drove around town until they found the other nurses who were still at work vaccinating and divided up the list of remaining houses with them. After several more hours, around midnight, Bill, Laura, and the nurses assisting them finished their rounds of the entire communities of Elizabethtown and New Russia. They counted 25 smallpox victims, with half of them nearly dead. Bill's sense of foreboding mounted with each new victim. He did his best to console the family members and comfort the ill. As the group was pulling into the hospital parking lot, Bill heard the familiar beating sound of helicopter rotors.

"Do you hear that?" he asked.

"Yes," answered Laura. "A helicopter?"

"Sounds like a Blackhawk. I wonder what's going on." They jumped out of the vehicle and scanned the sky. "It reminds me of my Army time when I bunked next to the flight line - they make a distinct sound because of the combination of the main rotor and the two powerful engines. Sounds a bit like an eggbeater on steroids."

"There," Laura said, pointing to a flashing red light in the sky above the school. The Blackhawk was about 1000 feet up and descending rapidly.

"It's landing in the soccer field. Let's go." They hopped back into the car and sped over to the school. By the time they reached the field, the Blackhawk was hovering about 100 feet in the air with the landing lights on.

Bill and Laura got out of the car, but turned their faces away, as the rotor wash from the chopper nearly knocked them over, and dust and debris swirled all around them. The

Blackhawk landed and the sound of the beating rotors slowly wound but didn't stop.

"You wait here," Bill yelled. He ducked his head low and ran around to approach from the rear of the chopper, just as the side door slid open. Four men dressed like aliens in plastic orange suits, clear plastic bubble hoods, green boots, and yellow gloves stepped out in slow motion. The noise from the engine was so loud that Bill couldn't understand what they were saying. He motioned for them to follow him away from the chopper. When they reached a comfortable distance, Bill stood upright again.

"I'm Dr. Denton," Bill yelled.

"Colonel Seeslack," the tall bald man said, his voice muffled by the plastic hood, "medical director of the Aeromedical Isolation Team. We're from USAMRIID. Sorry I can't shake your hand." He gestured toward his colleague standing behind him. "I believe you know Colonel Martinez."

In the dim light, Bill hadn't recognized his old friend, whose familiar jet-black hair and mustache from just a few years ago were now snowy white.

"Son of a bitch! Martinez!"

Martinez smiled. "Hey old buddy. Glad to see you're still with us. I'd give you a bear hug, but it's against regulations."

"That's okay. I'm glad to see you, too."

"We're here to take that frozen body off your hands," Martinez said. "In the last several hours, a lot has changed. The medical folks from CDC and USAMRIID have talked some sense into the other crisis players around the DC Beltway. The pattern of spread of the outbreak could be explained by natural means, without implicating terrorism, but the key to the proof is getting some virus from that body – as you suggested in your email."

"Wow!" Bill swore. "So, my last email got through after all?"

"Sure did. Can't say I would've thought about it

otherwise. My commander made a few phone calls to grease the skids, and here we are. We brought our mobile isolation unit to collect that body so we can study it further. Can you find us a pick-up truck?"

"Okay," Bill said. "The body's in the morgue. Give me a couple minutes."

"I'll come with you," Martinez said. He turned to his colleague. "Colonel Seeslack, you hang here with the rest of the team."

Bill and Laura drove Martinez over to the hospital, where they borrowed a truck from one of the nurses. Laura stayed behind at the hospital while Bill drove back to the chopper with Martinez.

Martinez's suit had a portable, battery-powered air filter attached to his back, which made a humming sound, so Bill had to raise his voice for Martinez to hear.

"What's the latest from the outside world?" he yelled.

"Everything's still mayhem, although there are some hopeful signs of progress. The CDC's starting to track down the cases. They've been augmented by state and county health department folks, as well as the Operational Medicine guys at USAMRIID. Half the battle is determining which leads are real and which are rumors. Lots of worried well are inundating hospitals, which has been compounded by desertions among the medical staff."

"Yeah," Bill said, "I'm familiar with that."

"Despite all the preparedness efforts in the past few years, people are still scared to death they'll catch something, even if they're vaccinated. The media's been using mass information campaigns across the country, and it seems to be having some effect. The exodus from east coast cities has led to some major gridlock. The National Guard's starting to make a dent, but they're pretty jumpy as well. There have been some shootings of unruly mobs."

"What about the vaccine?"

"They've begun to release some lots of the vaccine

that had been hoarded for the military. This has helped ease the vaccine crunch for targeting high-risk groups. Local law enforcement and the FBI are hoping to round up some of the vaccine thieves, but we're still under martial law. Any movement is challenging right now."

"Sounds a lot like what happened here. Once we established some control, things improved quickly. What about the rest of the world?"

"Things are still pretty tense. The President's had a couple emergency calls with other heads of state. As much as they want to cordon us off, they've begun to realize that if they don't help us quell this thing, they'll have their own problems. There are about 50 million doses of the vaccine elsewhere around the globe, so the CDC and the World Health Organization have enlisted various countries to donate a portion of their vaccine stockpiles to the hot spots with verified smallpox cases. The North Koreans seemed to back off on their doomsday rhetoric once we started to restore order."

"Damn!" Bill swore. "Amazing what a few hours can do."

Bill pulled the truck up to about 50 feet from the Blackhawk. The AIT members carried their seven foot-long clear plastic isolation unit out of the chopper and put it on the back of the pick-up.

Bill drove the team to the hospital, where they placed the frozen body into the isolator.

"Where are you taking him?" Bill asked on the drive back to the school field.

"USAMRIID. We've got the only BSL-4 maximum containment morgue in the country," Martinez said, "which has direct access into the laboratory. We'll put him to bed there until we can analyze some samples. After that, who knows? We'd like to characterize this virus and determine why it caused so many people to get hemorrhagic smallpox rather than the more common forms. We also might learn a thing or two about preserving life forms, given its long survival in the permafrost."

Once back at the field, Bill got out of the truck and watched the team load the isolator into the side of the Blackhawk. He had one last glimpse of the frozen body inside the plastic carrier before it was loaded up into the Blackhawk. The taut gray skin was barely visible in the dim light. His mocking half-smile seemed to suggest he had his own private joke. Who was that man? What had happened to him? Bill only knew that he met a horrific end, no different than Jeremy and others. So much had changed since Norm had first called him about the body.

Martinez approached Bill after the body was loaded.

"Well, buddy, you can't imagine the good you've done for the country. If the virus in this body matches the one isolated from Felicia Jamison, then you've saved us all a witch-hunt for phantom bioterrorists who don't exist. Oh, I almost forgot. The CDC director asked me to give you this - with his compliments." Martinez placed something cold in Bill's palm. "Stay safe. Let's get together when this is all over."

Martinez saluted Bill and then followed the others under the rotor and into the side door of the Blackhawk. Bill waved as Martinez pulled the Blackhawk door closed and the beating of the main rotor increased. He braced himself against the truck, turned his head, and closed his eyes as the rotor kicked up the dust around him and the wind pummeled his back. As the wind eased, he turned around to watch the Blackhawk ascend. He felt a final blast of air as the chopper headed south. Within seconds, it was gone and the immediate surroundings were quiet – as if it had never even been there. The cacophony elsewhere in the town returned, as he heard again horns honking and yelling.

After the lights of the chopper disappeared into the clouds, Bill hurried back to the truck. He needed to move quickly, in case some curious onlookers, drawn by seeing the helicopter, arrived at the field. He could barely see what the cold object was in his palm that Martinez had handed to him. He flipped a switch to turn on the truck's interior light. In the dim lighting he saw in his palm a vial containing a white powder and a syringe with a small amount of liquid. The vial label read: *Dryvax*. He couldn't believe it. His mind filled with images of all the suffering patients he'd seen in the last two days. It was amazing how priceless such a small vial could be. In his palm there was enough vaccine to contain any more cases that might occur, if he used it judiciously. Since he'd already variolated those at highest risk, he could now expand the target population to further decrease the risk of spread, since the vaccine was safer than variolation. Hot tears poured down his cheeks as he sobbed with relief. It was over.

38

Two Weeks Later

"To our friendship," Bill said as he lifted his wineglass. Bill, Martinez, Laura, and Nettie all sat around the kitchen table in Bill's father's house and lifted their wineglasses in tandem.

"I have to hand it to you all," Martinez said. "You've really done the nation, and the world, a service. If you guys hadn't blown the whistle on the re-emergence the world's most deadly scourge, which used to be nicknamed the 'most terrible of all the ministers of death,' it might have taken another week to know what was happening. By then, this monster would have spread even farther than it has already. Or worse yet, we'd still be going down the wrong path on a witch hunt for bioterrorists."

"We don't deserve the credit," Bill protested. "My dad was the key. He suspected it first, but he never got the chance to tell us."

"Maybe so, but your response with quarantine and variolation probably saved this town. Things were desperate, and you did the best you could with what you had."

"Well," Bill said, "you gave me the tools to run an outbreak investigation, and we just used the surveillance and containment model from the global eradication effort as our guide. I owe a debt of gratitude to my history professor over here." Bill squeezed Laura's hand. She smiled back and blushed.

"When all is said and done," Martinez said, "this one will definitely make it into the history books."

"You know, Bill," Nettie remarked with a mischievous grin, "with the mayor resigning due to his horrible incompetence and after losing his wife, we have a position open. I've heard your name mentioned as a possible candidate."

"No thanks, Nettie," Bill answered with a chuckle. "I'll stay within my comfort zone. If you need a town doctor instead, I might be willing to entertain an offer, as long as I get to pick a competent nurse." Bill winked at Laura. "Even if Rosemary survives her bout with smallpox, I could never trust her again after what she pulled stealing that vaccine."

"Don't worry," said Nettie. "I'm sure we can come up with an appropriate compensation package: friendly patients, occasional food from the neighbors, beautiful mountain scenery –"

"Don't forget the hospitable postwoman," Laura said.

"Definitely," Nettie said. "Well, with that said, it's time for this old postwoman to go home. The mail starts again tomorrow. No doubt there's a lot backed up. I may have dodged smallpox, but my arthritis is killing me." Nettie got up from the table and they all exchanged goodbyes.

After Nettie left, Laura said, "I don't want to put a damper on the evening, but I'm going to turn in as well."

"You okay?" Bill reached over and squeezed her hand.

Laura put her other hand on her forehead. "I'm starting to get a headache. I think I need to lie down."

Bill studied her face closely. Her flushed cheeks concerned him. "You don't have a fever, do you?"

"I'm fine." She patted his hand. "My face always turns red when I drink wine. You two enjoy the evening. You've got a lot of catching up to do." She got up from the table and put her dishes in the sink. She came back and kissed Bill on the forehead and whispered in his ear. "See you…later." His ear tickled as she blew on it lightly.

Bill watched Laura walk down the hall and prayed she wasn't getting ill. She said she'd never been vaccinated as a child, which was surprising, since she barely had any reaction to the variolation he gave her. Without an adequate response, she could still be susceptible and within the time window to develop smallpox from the recent exposures. Her headache could be the first symptom. He decided not to stay up too late, just to keep an eye on her.

"So, what's going to happen now?" Bill asked, as he turned his attention back to Martinez.

"So far, smallpox has been confirmed in 35 states and 30 countries. In the past week we've started to get some hopeful signals, with the rate of new infections cut by 50%. The government's looking at how we can crank out more vaccine quickly – possibly in the old way, by injecting virus onto the bellies of calves and then later harvesting the lymphatic fluid. In some places, they're using arm-to-arm vaccination: once one person develops a pustule from the vaccine, we'll use that fluid to vaccinate others in their family." Martinez fiddled with his bushy mustache. "One of the advantages we have now that we didn't have in the 1960's and 70's is my global Internet surveillance system. We can identify and squelch a pocket of disease around the globe quicker than before. It's going to take some time – maybe a couple months, maybe even as long as a year, but we're going to bury this disease again."

"It's incredible that this all started from a single frozen body," Bill remarked. He got up from the table. "You want some more wine?"

"Sure, but only half a glass."

Bill poured Martinez and himself more wine before returning to the table. He took a deep breath and savored the chocolaty aroma mixed in with hints of cherry and oak.

"Just shows how vulnerable our society is now," Martinez said as he picked up his mug, "with large metropolitan centers, mass transit, and air travel."

"Yeah. Can't get away from it," Bill said.

"By the way," Martinez said, "they finally found the specimen that your colleague, Norm, sent. It got lost in transit somewhere en route to the CDC from the New York State Health Department. Some of the workers in the original lab in

Saranac Lake and the reference lab in Albany came down with smallpox shortly after working with the sample. Fortunately, the DNA in the virus from that frozen body that Norm sent matched the virus that USAMRIID extracted from the body and also the virus from Felicia Jamison. That gave me ammunition to call off the hunt for bioterrorists."

"I'm glad," said Bill, "but don't we need to be concerned that someone might unleash smallpox again in the future as a weapon – especially now that nature's reminded us how devastating it can be?"

"Believe me," Martinez answered, shaking his head and opening his eyes wide. "That's the kind of thing that keeps me up at night, especially since labs all around the world now have samples. At the very least, we'll need to maintain some vaccine in storage. So, what are your plans now?"

Bill leaned back in his chair and sipped his wine. The warmth of the wine felt good in his chest, because the sun had set long ago, sending a chill throughout the house. "I never thought I'd admit it, but the work these past several weeks has been some of the most exciting I've ever done. I've always loved it here, but I never thought I'd like being the town doc. It's a lot different running the show myself, rather than working as second fiddle to my dad. I'm leaning pretty strongly towards staying. I've proposed to my colleagues in Washington, DC to use the clinic here as a rural training site for medical students from our affiliate schools. They could spend a month rotation here with me to get a taste of rural medicine. I think it's going to happen. This way, I get to maintain my link to an academic center."

"That's great," Martinez said. "I hope it works out. I really appreciate your invitation to come here and review the data on your inoculation effort. It could be very valuable, especially since there was such a high percentage of victims here with hemorrhagic smallpox. You cut the death rate down to about one-third of what it could have been. They'll be studying this outbreak and this strain of the virus for years. My buddies at USAMRIID already have a whole bunch of research proposals lined up.

Martinez leaned back in his chair and his mood lightened. "You know, that Laura is something else. If I were you, pal, I'd hold onto her." Martinez grinned while giving Bill a friendly punch on the arm.

“Yes. She’s a big part of why I want to stay. In fact, I should check on her. I might as well turn in too."

"I don't blame you, buddy," Martinez winked.

"Laura set up my Dad's old room for you. She's sanitized it well, but just in case, when was your last smallpox vaccine?"

"Don’t worry,” said Martinez. “I was vaccinated a couple years ago when I investigated a monkeypox outbreak in Africa. I wouldn't have been bold enough to come up here if I hadn't been. By the way, I’ll probably head out tomorrow – gotta help the WHO kill this outbreak with my surveillance network."

"Okay. See you in the morning before you go."

Bill’s footsteps echoed off the wooden floor as he walked down the hall and climbed the stairs cautiously. He feared the worst for Laura. Could she have a fever by now? As he reached the top of the stairs, he had a terrible vision of Laura covered with pustules. He didn’t think he could bear to witness such a horrible transformation.

He tiptoed into her bedroom. The room was dark. As the door slowly squeaked open, a sliver of light crept up to the bed. It was empty. Surprised, he left and walked over to his room. The small reading light next to his bed was on, but still no Laura. Standing in the doorway puzzled, he caught a whiff of her perfume and nearly jumped as her arms enveloped his waist.

"Don't move. You're mine."

He reached down and felt Laura's tiny hands before turning around. Her black hair shined in the dim light, and her dark eyes looked up at him longingly. She wore a silky white chemise, which ended just above her knees. He reached behind her and ran his finger down her spine as their lips met in a deep kiss. He moved his lips to her cheek and then her ear, while whispering, "I thought you weren't feeling well."

"I just wanted to get ready for you," she whispered back with a giggle. "Do you like it?" She twirled in front of him, lifting the edge of the chemise to reveal her pink French cut panties. He grabbed her and moved his hand down to her buttock and squeezed.

"I love it, but wouldn't this be considered sexual harassment?" he joked.

"Not if its consensual," she whispered, and gave him another kiss. "Besides, I'm no longer taking care of your father, so there's no issue."

As Bill massaged Laura's left thigh and hip, his hand stopped over a large irregular bump on her upper thigh.

"No. Please, don't touch that." She pulled his hand away.

"What? Why? Don't worry. I just want to take a look." Laura reluctantly sat down on edge of the bed, while Bill re-placed his hand on her thigh and his fingers explored the quarter-sized undulating surface and irregular border.

Laura leaned head back onto the pillow, her hair flowing outward. "It happened when my mother took me to Taiwan when I was a girl. I don't remember how I got it, but I hate it. Kids used to tease me when I wore a bathing suit in the summer. Can't you just ignore it?" she pleaded.

Bill leaned over to take a closer look. Suddenly he fell back on the bed, laughing.

Laura jumped up off the bed. "I know it's ugly," she said, "but you don't have to laugh about it." Tears streaked down her cheeks.

Bill grabbed her hand and gently pulled her back onto the bed. "That's not why I'm laughing. Don't you realize? That's a smallpox vaccine scar. You *were* vaccinated before after all."

"Really? I don't understand."

"There's no doubt. At one point, they vaccinated girls on their upper thighs, because they thought the scar would be less visible. That was before bikinis. I was so worried you might not have adequate immunity, because you hardly reacted to the variolation I gave you. But now I realize the reason your reaction was so mild was because you probably still have leftover immunity, especially with such a strong previous reaction. I'm laughing from relief. You can't imagine how much. Come here."

He gave her a strong hug. "I'm falling in love with you, Laura. I would never laugh at you. It's just that I was worried about you, and all along, there was probably no need."

She hugged him back and kissed him again.

39

Bill awoke suddenly. He reached over and felt Laura's warm body snuggled up next to him. She was still asleep, but something had awakened him and put him on edge. Then he heard it – heavy footsteps climbing slowly up the stairs. He got out of bed and made it to the doorway in time to see Henry O'Donnell stepping onto the second-floor landing.

"Henry," Bill called as he moved into the hallway, "what the hell are you doing here?"

"I'm here for retribution. You should have saved my wife. You're going to pay for her death."

"What are you talking about?" Bill protested. "I did everything I could to save her, but smallpox got her very quickly. She was a casualty like so many others – and your actions didn't help the situation."

"Don't blame me, you bastard," Henry said, as he hoisted his shotgun and leveled it at Bill's chest. Henry was now about 10 feet away from Bill. A blast this close would surely kill him.

"Henry, are you crazy? What do you think you're doing? Cold blooded murder won't bring your wife back. You'll go to prison and never see the light of day."

Henry's mouth twisted into a sickening grin. "You see, doc, that's the funny thing. I really don't care. You robbed me of everything I cared about – my wife, my job, and even the hotel I was building. I don't have anything more to live for."

Henry's gaze shifted slightly. Bill sensed why. Laura had awakened and was now standing behind him in the doorway.

"Well, isn't that convenient," Henry said. "I'm going to get a twofer – you *and* your girlfriend."

"Don't be an idiot, Henry. Laura's done you no harm.

Leave her out of this." Bill waved his arm. "Laura, get back in the room. Don't come out."

"At one point, years ago, I thought you were one of us," Henry said, "but now you're a city boy. You don't belong here anymore, and since you won't leave, I'm going to take care of that – for everyone."

While Henry was talking, Bill noticed movement in his peripheral vision. Martinez had entered the hall quietly downstairs. Bill didn't dare look in that direction, lest Henry became aware that Martinez was there. He needed to stall Henry as long as possible.

"Henry, everyone has something to live for. Your sister, Rosemary might recover – even with your wife gone, you're not alone."

"Nice try, doc, but to be honest, I never really liked Rosemary. She was always the pampered one. I was stuck with all the responsibility."

"There must be something you still care about."

"Not really. You've had enough time, Doc. Do you have any last words, before you meet your maker?" Henry taunted.

Bill could see that Martinez had pulled one of his father's spears off the wall. Martinez wound his arm back like a spring, ready to launch the spear.

"Yes, I do," said Bill, calmly.

"And? Let's hear it." asked Henry.

"NOW MARTINEZ." Bill dove for the floor just as Martinez uncoiled his arm and let the spear fly. The shotgun blast peppered the wall with spray just as the spear caught Henry in the side of his chest, slicing between his ribs and into his right lung. Henry gasped as he dropped the shotgun and fell to the ground, while blood spurted from his chest. Martinez ran up the stairs and jumped on Henry, pinning him down. Henry gasped for breath as blood sprayed out onto the floor. Laura threw Bill a towel and he rushed over to Martinez, where he applied pressure around the spear to stem the bleeding, but he didn't remove the spear, because it could cause more bleeding inside Henry's chest. Laura ran to the telephone upstairs and called for an ambulance. Next, she called the sheriff. The entire event couldn't have lasted more than five minutes.

Henry was adequately subdued but still having difficulty breathing by the time the ambulance arrived with a paramedic, and the medical team was accompanied by two deputy sheriffs.

"He's probably got a collapsed lung with a tension pneumothorax," Bill said to the medic. "Air pressure is building up inside his chest. Hand me a large bore needle."

The medic handed Bill a needle and he slowly inserted it into the upper part of Henry's right chest. There was a loud hissing sound as air pressure escaped Henry's chest, and his breathing eased. "He should be good until he gets to the hospital," Bill said to the medic. The ambulance left with Henry shortly thereafter, sirens blaring. One deputy accompanied the ambulance to guard Henry.

After Bill informed the other deputy about what had happened, he took statements from Bill, Martinez and Laura. "Don't worry, Doc," he said, "we'll make sure Henry can't do this again."

When the deputy left, Martinez asked, "Are you two okay?"

"Yes," said Laura, "but that was close."

"Yeah," said Bill, "and that makes three times in the past couple weeks that someone has threatened me with a shotgun."

"Hopefully three is enough," Laura said, as she wrapped her arms around Bill.

"By the way, Martinez," Bill said, "I was thinking about redecorating and removing my father's African art. It's a good thing I didn't yet. That spear sure came in handy. Where the hell did you learn to throw a spear like that. I know they didn't teach you that in the Army."

"Ha ha," Martinez laughed. "Definitely not. I threw the javelin on the high school track team – I was even the state champion. You never know when something like that will come in handy. Now that I'm awake, even though it's still dark out, I think I'll get ready to head back to Washington – before anything else crazy happens in this town."

"I don't blame you," Bill responded. "I don't think I could go back to sleep after what just happened. I know that Joel Brown is on call in the ER tonight, so he'll probably stabilize Henry and ship him off if he needs his chest cracked for internal repair, but I'm going to shower and dress anyway. I'd like to go to the hospital to personally ensure that Henry gets taken somewhere to fix him – both physically *and* mentally, so we don't have something like this happen again."

"I'm coming with you," Laura said.

40

The door creaked as Norm Phinney squeezed his heavy frame into the morgue. The place still retained the acrid stench of paraformaldehyde after a special government decontamination team had removed all the bodies and then fogged the lab interior. Norm flicked on the lights and lumbered over to his desk and sat down. He still felt a residual dull throb at his temples from the concussion caused by the car crash. He reluctantly started to sort through the stack of mail that awaited him on his desk from his week of recovery.

Norm felt somewhat disappointed that all the excitement was over. The scar on his finger had reached its final stage of healing but retained a slight pink tinge around the edges. He rubbed it a couple times, thankful that he'd been protected from smallpox by a quirk of fate.

He got up from his desk and walked over to the freezer. The red numbers on the digital temperature gauge read *-80 degrees*. The government team had left his freezer untouched. He donned a HEPA filter mask, gown, and insulated gloves before opening the freezer. Mist flowed out around the opening as he reached in and pulled out a tiny vial.

Even with the gloves on, the chill of the vial crept through to his fingers. He scraped off some ice on the vial and held it up to the light. The label read only *John Doe* with the date the frozen body was discovered at the Ice Cave. It contained a small piece of human tissue and about a thimble-full of frozen liquid. Norm carried it over to the sink and turned on the faucet. The water gurgled down the drain as he waited for it to warm up so he could melt the specimen and dump it into the sink. He doubted smallpox virus could survive with the other organisms competing in the sewer system. Before melting the specimen, he held the frozen vial up one last time and rotated it in the light. There was something beautiful about the perfect killing power of the microscopic life forms inside that vial – frozen again in time, as they had been for over five decades. Nature had created a microbe equivalent of the atomic bomb.

"Idiot!" he chastised himself, suddenly realizing that he was staring at pure gold. It might not be worth much now, but maybe in five or ten years, when all the excitement about smallpox died down, the world would be declared free of smallpox again. Countries around the globe would stop vaccinating. When that happens, the billions of tiny virus particles imprisoned inside the vial could be worth millions. Their ability to kill and maim had already been demonstrated with thousands of victims worldwide. Someone, perhaps a rogue nation or a terrorist organization, could be very interested. Why not profit from it? If he just sold it to someone, it wasn't his fault if they released it, was it? He would just be supplying a product, just like any business transaction.

Satisfied with this logic, Norm walked quickly back across the room, cradling his newfound investment and placed it gingerly back in the freezer.

Epilogue

March 1947

The traveler climbed over the last few boulders to reach the summit of Lower Wolfjaw Mountain's undulating peak. Snow from the night before still blanketed the dwarfed shrubs that surrounded him as he stepped through snow up to his mid-shins. The winter had been mild; otherwise, the snow at this level would have been several feet deeper. A crisp blue sky above him was like a canvas, brushed with only a few scattered wisps of clouds above mist-shrouded valleys and jagged mountains.

The traveler's connection to the Adirondack mountains began during childhood summer vacations, when he would gaze at the stars while his father entertained him with stories of the Native Americans who settled the picturesque region. He had always wanted to return as an adult to climb the mountains and leave the tourist valleys below. Now approaching 30, with his fair skin showing its first wrinkles and his sandy hair sporting premature strands of gray, the traveler had spent the past two weeks in and out of smoke-filled bus stations with crying babies, toothless old men, and vagabonds with rank body odor. His route took him up from Mexico to Indianapolis, on to New York City, then north to the Adirondacks. During the final stretch of the journey, the bus bounced over narrow dirt mountain roads into the town of Elizabethtown, population: 250. He used the town as his launching point for a series of hikes into the surrounding High Peaks region. He spent most of the day climbing over a series of foothills en route to mountain number 10, called Gothics, which was now visible off in the distance, its pointed peak towering above him like a Gothic cathedral.

After finishing an apple and enjoying the

breathtaking scenery, the traveler knew night would fall soon, and he needed to find a sheltered area to prepare for the night's cold. He hoisted his backpack and picked his way through the snowpack and undergrowth down into the final dip below Gothics. As he made his way down the slope, occasionally sliding on ice patches, he ignored twinges of flu-like aches in his joints and muscles, assuming they must be the price for the rigorous climbing.

A two-story granite wall covered with a thin sheet of ice provided a sheltered place to set up camp. Some downed trees and boulders offered further protection from the chilling night wind. He set about collecting pine boughs to make his bed, and then he gathered some twigs for a fire. As the shadows lengthened around him, he huddled close to the fire, enjoying the military rations he brought, which tasted surprisingly good after the exhausting day.

Periodic muscle twinges made him wonder whether he might have caught an illness during the trip. He remembered one gray suit, in particular, who sat across the aisle from him on the bus ride from Mexico north into the United States. The man's face was flushed cherry red and shined from a sheen of sweat. Periodically, his body shook violently before he let out a deep, wet cough. With each cough, the businessman had spewed millions of tiny particles that floated on the air currents around every passenger. The traveler's lungs sucked them in with his next couple of breaths, where they landed on a warm, moist area on the back of his throat suitable for microbial growth.

The traveler snuffed out the fire with some snow, then reclined on his bed of pine boughs, unaware of the battle raging inside his body against a foreign invader. He cocooned himself in his down sleeping bag and peered out into the night. The moonlight peaked through the canopy of evergreens above, leaving scattered patches of light on the granite wall next to him that danced as the trees swayed from the breeze.

Around midnight, he awoke suddenly as his body

convulsed with a violent, uncontrollable shiver. A stabbing pain pierced his back as sweat poured from his body, soaking his clothing and sleeping bag. His skin felt like hot embers, so he knew he must have a fever, but he'd never felt so deathly ill before. He rummaged through his backpack in the dark, with sweat-drenched hands and managed to find his canteen. He drank the water in great gulps, but then he wondered if drinking it had been a mistake. The water came from a stream he drank out of the day before – could that have made him sick? He shivered through the rest of that night praying for a quick recovery, but as the night led to another day and night of fever, he became less aware of his surroundings. During a lucid moment he prayed that he might die to end the misery.

On the third day, the fever finally subsided enough for him to sit up. His mouth was parched, with his tongue like sandpaper. Although he felt somewhat better, the invaders continued to multiply inside him, steadily destroying his vital organs. Fluid began to ooze into his lungs, causing him to cough and use more energy to take in each breath. His bowels began to slough their lining, allowing blood to trickle into his intestines. One by one, his brain cells exploded, numbing his senses, his emotion, and rational thought. In the dullness of his mind, his instincts deep down urged him to get down from the mountain to find water.

He stumbled from his pine bed, abandoning his equipment in a frantic pursuit of water. Wandering aimlessly down the mountain, he barely noticed the cold, only aware that his head pounded with explosive pain each time he coughed. Somewhere in the fog of his mind, he knew he was dying, but he struggled on, with a primitive fight to live. Eventually he stumbled out of the underbrush into a clearing, but his brain had difficulty registering the blurred image of a lake before him. Most of the lake appeared covered with ice, with a blanket of snow on top.

With great effort, he crawled to the edge and found a spot where some ice had melted, and he felt the cool water soothe his burning face. Taking in great gulps of water, some went down his windpipe, making him choke and cough. With each cough, something inside his chest ripped, but he could no longer feel the pain. He stared numbly at pools of blood and floating bits of tissue, not comprehending that he'd coughed them up. An apparition reflecting in the rippling water had large red and purple bruises and scattered tiny bumps where pockets of blood and pus had separated patches of skin on his face from the tissue beneath. The whites of both his eyes were now bright crimson. He tried to scream, but could only produce a gurgling sound, as he stumbled away from the water, horrified by the ghastly image.

He instinctively crawled like a beast toward the low pitch of a foghorn-like sound coming from a nearby cave, responding as if he were being summoned. He hoped he could find shelter to rest, but with each movement, his energy drained further. His muscles froze from lack of blood and the nerves controlling his movement short-circuited from the brain. In one great convulsion, his bowels opened and released gushes of blood mixed with his intestinal lining. The warm blood felt comforting, like swimming in amniotic fluid, as it poured down his pant-legs. He collapsed in an icy ditch, where a cool mist floated out of the cave into the ditch and enveloped him, soothing his fiery skin. He also felt relief as freezing rain and ice crystals landed on his face from a coming storm. The last thing he knew before losing consciousness was the pungent, raw, meaty stench of his own death.

The End

Notes From The Author

[Smallpox] was always present, filling the churchyard with corpses, tormenting with constant fear all whom it had not yet stricken, leaving on those whose lives it spared the hideous traces of its power, turning the babe into a changeling at which the mother shuddered, and making the eyes and cheeks of the betrothed maiden objects of horror to the lover.
T.B. Macaulay,
The History of England from the Accession of James II.

The Traveler

A real smallpox outbreak took place in 1947 in New York City. The first case in the United States was a businessman, Mr. Eugene Le Bar, who carried the disease on a bus from Mexico. During that outbreak, which resulted in 12 cases and 2 deaths, the New York City Health Department vaccinated over six million people over a couple days - an amazing feat. Old newspaper photographs show orderly lines of people several blocks long waiting for their vaccinations. When health officials tracked down all the people who Mr. Le Bar may have exposed, they had already scattered to 29 different states. It is conceivable that an unrecognized case, like the Traveler, could have been missed. Just imagine the global implications if a similar situation occurred now, given modern air travel, the limited number of people previously vaccinated, and new skepticism towards vaccines. The outbreak investigation would become a worldwide race against time to track down potential victims, much like what occurred in the 2003 SARS and 2020 SARS-CoV2 pandemics. There has been speculation that a lone terrorist could board a plane at his or her most contagious period and thus start a worldwide epidemic.

The Ice Cave

An ice cave that served as the inspiration for this story exists in a remote region of the Adirondack Mountains on private land on the lower Ausable Lake. The cave is made up of a large group of boulders. Snow during the winter falls behind them and is protected from the sun. In the summer, the air flowing down the mountain blows behind the boulders, over the protected snow and ice, and onto the lake, producing a cool mist. The temperature of the surrounding air and water is noticeably cooler than the rest of the lake all year round.

Smallpox

Variola, the scientific name of the smallpox virus, comes from the Latin *varius*, meaning "spotted" or "stained." Compared with other devastating diseases of antiquity, including anthrax, tuberculosis, cholera, plague, and polio, smallpox has arguably had the most persistent and universal impact on the human species. It affected the royalty as well as the poor. At one time, any human born into this world was destined to meet smallpox, and they would either live or die.

I first conceived the idea to write this book in 1995 while taking a class on outbreak investigation at the Harvard School of Public Health. My professor, Jonathan Freeman, commented that even though smallpox had been eradicated, there was probably a laboratory somewhere in the world with a forgotten, unlabeled vial of smallpox virus in the back of a freezer. He postulated that someday someone might take an unlabeled vial out, expose themselves, and inadvertently start the next smallpox pandemic. At the time, neither my professor nor I realized how prescient his notion was, given the concerns that surfaced later about smallpox as a potential bioterrorist weapon. In 2014, unsecured vials containing smallpox virus were found in a freezer at the National Institutes of Health in Bethesda, Maryland.

The eradication of smallpox was one of the greatest public health triumphs of all time. After the eradication, the

World Health Organization requested all countries around the globe to either destroy or turn in their smallpox samples to central repositories in the United States and the former Soviet Union. Currently there remain only two known legal stores of live smallpox virus at the Centers for Disease Control and Prevention in Atlanta and the State Research Center of Virology and Biotechnology, Koltsovo, Russian Federation. There continues to be speculation that additional specimens may have been retained in other laboratories around the world and that victims of smallpox buried in the Siberian permafrost could provide the seeds for an outbreak. Dr. Ken Alibek, former deputy director in the civilian arm of the Soviet biological weapons program, *Biopreparat*, revealed that the Soviets had the capability to produce metric tons of smallpox virus annually and at one point loaded it in intercontinental ballistic missiles aimed at major cities in the United States. This information raised smallpox to the top of the list of potential biological weapons that could be used for warfare or terrorism to cause mass casualties. Questions remain about what happened to all the smallpox produced and whether some of the former Soviet scientists may have been wooed to biological weapon programs in countries around the globe that sponsor terrorism.

Despite several planned dates of virus execution, the United States has decided not destroy its smallpox stores for the foreseeable future so more research can be done on the virus. The World Health Assembly subsequently followed suit. The virus therefore continues, alive, in suspended (frozen) animation at this time.

There continue to be arguments in favor of destroying and not destroying the virus. Those who want to destroy the virus are concerned about the possibility of accidental or intentional release. Others argue that some might view retaining the virus as legitimizing the retention of stockpiles of biological weapons. The argument is also made that research could be done on other similar viruses instead of

Variola, such as mpox or *Vaccinia*.

Those in favor of retaining the virus argue that there are unique properties of smallpox that must be studied since smallpox in the natural setting causes deadly disease only in humans. They also note that there are other potential sources already out there from cadavers in the permafrost or virus specimens lost in somebody's freezer, and that the sequence for the smallpox genome is already determined. Consequently, there are potential sources for an outbreak, and we therefore gain nothing from destroying the stocks of virus, whereas there are legitimate reasons for retaining the virus. Researchers at USAMRIID, in collaboration with the CDC, successfully induced disease in monkeys, opening the door for establishing a primate animal model in which potential treatments, such as cidofovir, could be tested. An antiviral product, Tecoviramat, was recently licensed for the treatment of smallpox. So, retention of the virus has already yielded potential benefits.

Regardless of which perspective one takes, or whether the formal destruction ever occurs, because of its potential to kill, blind, and disfigure humans, smallpox will continue to be a concern for bioterrorism and biowarfare. There will probably always be unease about undeclared or unknown stores of the virus. Interestingly, use of smallpox as a weapon occurred in the 1700s during the French and Indian War when a British officer, Sir Geoffrey Amherst, gave smallpox-contaminated blankets and handkerchiefs to Indians sympathetic to the French under the guise of "gifts." The smallpox vaccine is a very effective vaccine (after all, it helped eradicate the disease). Once the vaccine was developed, using smallpox as a weapon was no longer an issue – at least until we stopped vaccinating against it. Currently, a minority of the worldwide population would have any immunity to smallpox since routine vaccination stopped over 40 years ago.

The current U.S. stockpile of smallpox vaccine has

grown since an earlier version of this book was published in 2004. At that time, there were only 15.4 million doses. If one looks at the 1947 outbreak of smallpox in New York City, where over 6 million doses were used to stop the outbreak, a stockpile of 15.4 million doses is hardly adequate for the U.S. population in the event of a large outbreak. After the terrorist attacks of September 11, 2001, and the 2001 anthrax letter scare, the national stockpile numbers have increased to vaccinate the entire US population, if needed. President George W. Bush subsequently mandated smallpox vaccine for all U.S. forces and it was offered to select civilian health care professionals, but that effort ended abruptly due to concerns of side effects. Nonetheless, by having a store of vaccine available for use in case of an outbreak, one hopes a terrorist or military adversary would be deterred from using it. If it were used, the outbreak could ideally be brought under control quickly, but likely with some measure of chaos and disruption. Without a doubt, given the historical devastation smallpox has caused, it will always be a disease that strikes fear in the hearts of humans and has the potential to rise again, as it did in this novel in the small town of Elizabethtown, in upstate New York.

Even when smallpox was common, it was frequently confused with chickenpox until several days had passed. While finalizing production of a satellite program on the medical management of biological weapon casualties, I asked a dermatologist to watch one of our scenarios about a smallpox outbreak. Despite knowing the show's subject, the dermatologist didn't recognize the disease as smallpox. Clearly, we have a long way to go in re-educating our medical care providers on this deadly scourge that once was called the "most terrible minister of death." Would a lone practitioner today recognize a case of smallpox in time to make a difference even though it hasn't been seen in the United States for nearly 80 years? Hopefully we'll never know.

Mark Kortepeter, 2026

Smallpox Timeline

1796: Edward Jenner, a country doctor in England, reports that humans inoculated with cowpox are protected against smallpox. This information leads to the first protective vaccine.

1901-1903: The second to last major American smallpox epidemic (Boston, New York, Philadelphia). Death rate from the disease in 1901 was 18.4% of victims.

1920: Last major U.S. epidemic.

1947: Epidemic in New York City, imported by a businessman, Mr. Eugene Le Bar, traveling on a bus up from Mexico. Over 6 million persons were vaccinated in New York City to control the epidemic. Total cases of smallpox: 12. Total deaths: 2.

January 1, 1967: The World Health Organization launches the Intensified Smallpox Eradication Program. At this time 10-15 million cases of the disease were occurring every year in more than 30 countries. Up to two million died and millions were left blind or disfigured each year.

1971: Routine vaccination in the U.S. discontinued.

1976: Routine vaccination of health care workers discontinued.

October 1977: The last case of naturally acquired smallpox occurred in Somalia.

1978: British medical photographer, Janet Parker, died after exposure to laboratory smallpox through the ventilation system. Her mother was secondarily infected by her, but survived. The researcher whose lab caused the inadvertent exposure committed suicide.

May 1980: World Health Assembly certifies smallpox as eradicated.

1980: American College of Immunization Practice recommends smallpox vaccine for lab workers with potential exposure to vaccinia, mpox, and other orthopoxviruses.

January 1982: Smallpox vaccine no longer required for international travelers.

1982: Only active producer of vaccine in the U.S. discontinues production.

1983: Civilian smallpox vaccine distribution discontinued.

1992: Soviet defector Ken Alibek reveals the massive nature of the former Soviet bioweapons program, including the capability for producing metric tons of smallpox virus.

1995: Iraq admits to having conducted research on camelpox virus, a close relative to smallpox virus.

1997: Study published in the *Journal of Infectious Diseases* demonstrates the use of a new cell-culture-derived smallpox vaccine.

1999: President Clinton declares that the United States would not destroy its stocks of smallpox virus so that more research could be conducted.

2000: Research study conducted at St. Louis University to see whether the old Dryvax smallpox vaccine could be diluted 10 or 100-fold and still lead to adequate protection of the vaccinee. This would then allow the dilution of the limited U.S. stockpile of vaccine in a crisis and consequently would amplify the U.S. stockpile.

2000: U.S. military announces contract for production of 300,000 doses of vaccine. CDC announces a contract for 40 million doses for the national pharmaceutical stockpile. Both vaccines will be produced in cell culture, rather than the original method of production in calf lymph on live calves.

2001: Events of September 11 and anthrax contaminated letters prompt a re-evaluation of smallpox vaccine stockpile needs.

2002: The target date for the delivery of the first shipments of a new, cell-culture-derived smallpox vaccine. United Nations experts ask for a delay in the destruction of the remaining stocks of smallpox virus so that more research can be conducted on vaccines and treatments.

2003: Vaccine is offered to select civilian health care providers and ancillary health personnel.

Currently, the U.S. military vaccinates certain personnel based on exposure risk.

The questions remain – what other countries might still retain stores of the smallpox virus, and what happened to all the smallpox produced by the former Soviet Union's bioweapons program?

Selected References Used For This Book

Barquet N, Domingo P. Smallpox: the triumph over the most terrible of the ministers of death. *Annals of Internal Medicine* 1997. 127;8:635-42.

Benenson AS, Editor. Control of communicable diseases in man, 15th Ed. 1990. *American Public Health Association*, Washington, DC. 395-402.

Bowman L. Germ attack could be a pox on our houses. *The Sunday Journal*, March 14, 1999. A2.

Brown D. Destruction of smallpox samples is reassessed: some suspect virus also exists in secret. *The Washington Post*, March 15, 1999. A1.

Centers for Disease Control. Vaccinia (smallpox) vaccine: recommendations of the immunization practices advisory committee 1991. 40;RR-14: 1-10.

Fenner F, Henderson DA, Arita Z, Jezek, Ladnyi ID. Smallpox and its eradication. *World Health Organization* 1988. Geneva.

Gladwell M. The dead zone. *The New Yorker*, September 29, 1997. pp 52-58.

Infectious disease pathogens know no borders; surveillance will be key tool in coming battle. *The Nation's Health*, January 1997. pg. 20.

Okie S. U.S. to oppose destroying smallpox stocks: fears that virus is in wrong hands prompt shift unpopular with most of world. *The Washington Post*, April 23, 1999. A2.

Preston R. The bioweaponeers. *The New Yorker*, March 9, 1998. pp 52-65.

Sawyer K. Frozen mummies of Incas unearthed. *The Washington Post*, April 7, 1999. A1.

Smallpox Scare: New York vaccinates 2,000,000 for disease which might have spread through entire U.S. *Life Magazine*. 1947.

Acknowledgements

I am indebted to my former professor, Jonathan Freeman, who unknowingly gave me the idea for this book during an outbreak investigation class in 1995 while I was a student at the Harvard School of Public Health. I express my sincere gratitude to numerous other individuals who graciously spent time painstakingly reviewing the manuscript and providing me with their candid opinions and suggestions: Luann Engle, Dorothy Troup, Andrew Ragan, Sue Kremmer, Zyg Dembek, Cheryl Duke, Paul Kortepeter, and Patricia Petitt. I also appreciate others who read some of the manuscript or provided consultation on aspects of the manuscript: Aileen Marty, Karl Kortepeter, Jenny Kortepeter, Erica Kortepeter, Victor Bernet, and Howard Chazin. My colleagues Ed Eitzen, Scott Stanek, Ted Cieslak, and Ted Hussey also deserve my thanks for their encouragement and suggestions. I also want to thank my Harvard college professor, Harold Burzstajn, who taught a class on the uncertainty of medical decision making. During that class, he gave me latitude to write creatively. His encouragement inspired me to continue writing. I also appreciate the inspiration I have received from my parents, Max and Cynthia Kortepeter, who taught me that with persistence, anything is possible. In line with Thomas Edison's famous quotation that "Genius is 1% inspiration and 99% perspiration," I have learned that writing is more about drive and persistence than having a good story idea, although both are clearly required to bring a manuscript to fruition. Finally, I am most grateful to my wife, Cindy, who willingly endured with me through the whole process for the original book and all over again with this newly revised version. Her unvarnished opinions and critical eye for editing has improved everything I have written. And finally, to my children, Luke, Sean, and Daniel, who allowed my writing to steal time away from them.

About the Author

Dr. Mark G. Kortepeter is a physician, scientist, Army colonel (retired), and author. His career has spanned the hospital, research lab, the lecture hall, and the battlefield. Trained in infectious diseases and public health, with expertise in biological weapon defense, Dr. Kortepeter has held senior positions at the US Army Medical Research Institute of Infectious Diseases (USAMRIID), the Uniformed Services University, and the University of Nebraska Medical Center.

Dr. Kortepeter's medical thriller memoir, *Inside the Hot Zone: a Soldier on the Front Lines of Biological Warfare* (Potomac Books, 2020), details his experiences managing national infectious disease crises while at USAMRIID. It was a finalist for the 2021 William E. Colby Award and it was optioned for film/TV by CBS Studios. Kortepeter also served as a medical contributor on infectious disease and epidemic-related topics for *Forbes.com* from 2020-25.

www.ingramcontent.com/pod-product-compliance
Lightning Source LLC
LaVergne TN
LVHW090557110826
845146LV00001B/169

* 9 7 9 8 9 9 5 6 4 7 3 0 0 *